Nutrition From the Spirits

A Guide to Curing Illnesses as Dowsed From the Universal Force

Nutrition From the Spirits

A Guide to Curing Illnesses as Dowsed From the Universal Force

Ellen Engelkemier

iUniverse, Inc.
New York Lincoln Shanghai

Nutrition From the Spirits

A Guide to Curing Illnesses as Dowsed From the Universal Force

iUniverse books may be ordered through booksellers or by contacting:

iUniverse
2021 Pine Lake Road, Suite 100
Lincoln, NE 68512
www.iuniverse.com
1-800-Authors (1-800-288-4677)

ISBN: 978-0-595-47711-1 (pbk)
ISBN: 978-0-595-91973-4 (ebk)

Printed in the United States of America

This book is the result of over a thousand hours of dowsing. I believe that God gave me this information to put into a book that anyone could use. We do not have to be victums of ill health. God wants us to be well. We must take responsibility for maintaining our own health. My prayer is that people will use this book to cure themselves and loved ones. May we all learn to follow the guidance from within.

CONTENTS

Introduction

I began dowsing in 1998. While I experimented with dowsing for several things, I dowsed daily for nutrients to take. As I encountered various health problems, I relied on the advise of the pendulum to relieve or cure them. I had suspected that I had a thyroid problem as early as 1980. My skin would often remain cold even when I worked up a sweat. But doctors consistently told me I was wrong. In 2000, the fatigue had gradually increased to a point where I could barely get through a full work day. Each noon hour I would lie down in my pickup cab for at least 20 minutes, more if possible. Still, I was so tired I could barely function. I had heard that people got more tired as they grew older. How was I to know my fatigue was extreme? Finally, after quitting my job, I found it impossible to accomplish anything around home. Several times the fatigue hit so quickly and was so exhausting that I would have less than a minute before my legs gave out. My dowsing confirmed that the problem was thyroid. But it also told me that no doctor would prescribe thyroid for me because all my blood tests would be normal. I got great help from acupuncture but this was painful, expensive, and wore off after 6 months. I found a source of iodine and dowsed dosages to take. Eventually I was taking more than 80 times the Recommended Daily Allowance of iodine and I was still exhausted. After a year and a half, the pendulum finally directed me to a physician who confirmed my diagnosis through intuitive work. I got a prescription for thyroid. It took another two and a half years to reach the full dose of thyroid I need. I am now a strong and vibrant person more healthy than I have been in my life; I needed the thyroid since birth.

I had learned through dowsing that not only my relatives, but **15% of the U.S. population suffers from thyroid blockages** similar to mine. It occurred to me that my memory problems might be similar to early Alzheimer's symptoms or senile dementia. So I asked one night "Are some of the people suffering from Alzheimer's actually in need of thyroid like me?" The answer was "Yes". **"About what per cent of Alzheimer's patients would be okay if they took thyroid?"** The answer was "**80%**". My mouth dropped open. While the country fights about stem cell research and families spend hundred of dollars a month on drugs, 80% of these patients could be cured with $10 worth of thyroid!

I then dowsed about the remaining 20% of Alzheimer's patients only to learn that those patients have senile dementia and can be cured by taking vitamin E.

After getting this startling—if not shocking—information, I decided to go to bed. The hour was approaching midnight and I needed to digest this information. Additionally, I'd had a frustrating conversation that evening with a schizophrenic relative. In my lifetime I have had at least three relatives who suffered from schizophrenia: It is a terrible illness that causes suffering to the patient and everyone near the patient. If I could cure only one illness on this earth, it would not be Alzheimer's at least most of those patients are elderly. I would cure schizophrenia. So I was stunned but upset and crying that I didn't know how to help my loved one. "Well **what causes schizophrenia?**" I asked out loud. Words came to me. "**Lack of zinc mutates the collagen …**" That made zero sense to me. What would collagen have to do with the brain? I started thinking about all of the Alzheimer's patients in nursing homes who should be out living a good life instead. How could I help them? What should I do with the information I have? But the" zinc and collagen" thing kept coming back into my head. Finally, I got out of bed, turned on the light, and grabbed my copy of Balch and Balch.[1] I turned to the section that described minerals and flipped to "Zinc". The second sentence reads "It is required for protein synthesis and collagen formation …"[2] **There was no way I could have remembered any connection between collagen and zinc. I had been given the answer to my question.** Schizophrenia is (at least sometimes) caused by lack of zinc resulting in a mutation of collagen. I dowsed the question "Is there collagen in the brain?" "Yes".

That night, in the early hours of the morning, I dowsed for cures to schizophrenia, depression, and manic-depression before finally going to bed. I learned that the 'cure' to an illness is not necessarily indicative of the 'cause'. Sometimes the body lacks a nutrient that is necessary to utilize a second nutrient which cures the illness. I just want to see people healthy. I decided to dowse only for cures.

---

1. Prescription for Nutritional Healing, James F. Balch, M.D. and Phyllis A. Balch, C.N.C., 1990
2. Page 23, Prescription for Nutritional Healing, James F. Balch, M.D. and Phyllis A. Balch, C.N.C. 1990

Questions and Answers

If these illnesses can be cured by vitamins, minerals, etc., why can't we cure ourselves by just eating right?

One of the most important things we need to understand is that **we have to make up for missed dosages.** Perhaps as adult you eat a pretty balanced diet. But in your teenage years you may have tended to skip a lot of fruits and vegetables. At some point in your life you need to make up for each dose of vitamins, etc., that you missed, or the lack will result in an illness. In some cases, a person may actually need to make up for the nutrients which his/her mother missed before the person was born. By the time illness occurs, the deficiency is too great to make up by eating.

How can all these diseases be cured by nutrients if they are caused by viruses, insect bites, or other things in the environment?

Nutrients play many roles in our bodies. One of those roles is to defend us against attack from various environmental influences. Examples of this are things like the flu or anthrax. The people who do not succumb to these diseases, already have the necessary defense nutrients in their bodies.

In other cases, diseases are a direct result of malnutrition. To explain this, I like to use the analogy of a giant airplane that has hundreds of engines. Each engine requires a particular nutrient for fuel. Some may require several nutrients. When a particular engine runs out of 'fuel' it must shut down in an effort toward self preservation. That's the onset of a disease like diabetes or schizophrenia. Provide the right fuel and the engine can re-start.

Why is that the people who are unhealthy do not crave the foods which would help them?

There is a part of the brain that correlates to each nutrient the body needs. Once we get just so low on a particular nutrient, that part of the brain mutates and its receiver cannot get the correct message. The signals get misinterpreted. We begin to get signals that lack indication of the needed food. Instead, we get the craving for salt and sugar. This is why we wind up eating so much junk food.

If simple nutrients can cure these illnesses, why haven't physicians discovered it years ago?

Most medical researchers do not believe nutrition has that much to do with illness. If they do run tests with nutrients it is usually in very low doses and not enough to cure. The Universal Force informs me that through the years other people have dowsed for cures to illnesses and received the answers. But dowsing and other "paranormal" practices allowed the mass population to get well and individuals in power wanted to reduce the population. Therefore, such practices were ridiculed and sometimes even outlawed.

What about our emotions, thoughts, etc.… Don't they effect out health?

Absolutely! **Illness is caused 50% by malnutrition and 50% by wrong thinking!** If you suffer from a serious disease you may want to read books by Carolyn Myss and Mona Lisa Schultz. Both discuss how emotions and thought patterns effect the body. Ms Schultz is a medical doctor who has observed similar thought/beliefs among patients of same or similar diseases. Carolyn Myss is a mystic who sees illness within a person's body.

Getting well from a serious illness involves changing our outlook on the world. The Universal Force says that **serious illness is a call to become more spiritual.**

Why would God, the Universal Force or any other spirit choose YOU to give the answers to?

The answers are there for anyone who dowses.

It makes sense to me that balancing our bodies would not come from adding drugs foreign to the body but from increasing some nutrients that are natural to the body.

I have no medical background; I can accept this information. It does not oppose any previous conditioning that a medical person might have.

Many people would want to cure cancer and physical ailments but ignore mental illnesses.

Some physicians would not want the patient to have control over his or her treatment.

Where do answers come from when you dowse?

Every dowser might give a different answer to that question. I believe I get answers from different places. If I dowse to locate a misplaced item or for personal advice, I believe that my spirit guides often answer. When I began dowsing cures to illnesses, I asked where the answers were coming from and was told they come from the Universal Force. I believe the Universal Force is the melded consciousness of millions of persons who formerly lived on earth. The effect is like that of an incredibly giant computer.

My illness isn't listed in the book. Can I be cured or even helped?

Try to find someone in your area who dowses for nutrients. If you really cannot find anyone, you can copy and complete the form in the back of this book. Follow instructions given. An attempt will be made to dowse for special cases. Be forewarned—some people cannot be cured. This could be because the necessary nutrient is unavailable or because that person is not supposed to be healed. In all cases you will receive a reply.

I am embarrassed to tell people of the illness I have. If I ask for the nutrients in a health food store, will clerks know what it's for?

No. Every nutrient helps a variety of illnesses. But clerks often ask "What is it for?" thinking they might sell you something else if they don't have what you request. Be prepared to answer that question with "It's to treat a deficiency of (nutrient requested)".

Should a person stop taking prescription medications when using these treatments?

No. I would never tell you to ignore your physician's orders. The physician who prescribed the medication should determine when to discontinue it. Nutrients are condensed food. They should not interfere with other treatments.

Can I learn to dowse myself?

Sure! Most people are able to dowse. I do not recommend learning while you are recovering from a serious illness, but otherwise I think we should all dowse on a regular basis. I would suggest reading *Letter to Robin, A Mini-Course in Pendulum Dowsing* by Walt Woods. This is available via the American Society of Dowsers 1-802 684-3417 or www.asd@dowsers.org. It also helps to join a group if there is one in your area. Just be aware that you can get a lot of false reading if you are ill when dowsing.

Are nutrients affected by food preservation and preparation as canning, freezing, UV treated, Micro-wave, etc.?

Yes. Fresh is always best. Cooking on a stove with as little water as possible preserves more nutrients than heating in a microwave. Freezing preserves more nutrients than canning. Avoid UV treated foods; they have the least amount of nutrients.

Is there really any difference between the nutrition of organic food vs. conventionally grown food?

According to the Universal Force, the organic and conventionally grown foods have about the same nutritional values. Conventionally grown foods can also contain fertilizers and pesticides which tax our bodies' immune systems. It requires more nutrition to stay healthy eating conventional food than eating organic food.

Instructions for Using this Book

(Dowsers: Instructions for Using this Book via Dowsing are listed in back of book. *See* Index)

1. Read the information on Blocked Thyroid completely. Even if you do not have this problem, you may recognize symptoms that a loved one has.

2. Go through the listings of illnesses and mark every illness you experience with a bookmark. Now get a pen and paper. Begin with your most serious illness. List the Essential nutrient for that illness at the top of the piece of paper. This will be the first nutrient that you should take. If you take only the essential nutrient, you will be cured of that illness within the Maximum Cure Time. Below it, list all the Helpful items for that illness. Then turn to the next illness causing the most problem. Write down both the Essential and Helpful items for that illness. If an item listed is already on your page, put a mark beside it instead of writing it again. Continue doing this for every illness you experience no matter how serious or minor. When you have completed this process, you should have several marks next to certain nutrients. These are nutrients that you are seriously deficient in. Purchase and take these nutrients until cured of the most serious illnesses. Do not purchase or take more than five (5) different items at any one time. Put the list away and keep it. After curing your most serious illnesses, you may wish to work on other less serious illnesses at a later time.

Keep in mind that absolutely nothing makes up for a lack of thyroid. If you have a thyroid blockage, essential items may help but not cure serious illnesses.

Note: Many nutrients—especially amino acids and enzymes—may need to be purchased in combination with other supplements not necessarily indicated. This is fine so long as you dowse or muscle test to make certain no ingredients will give you an adverse reaction. READ CONTAINER LABELS. If directions are to take that pill before eating, with food, etc. FOLLOW DIRECTIONS. If you need to avoid grapefruit because of medicine you are taking, you should also avoid L-citruline, L-serine, L-taurine, bromeline, and vitamin C.

MUSCLE TESTING

At home with a friend, prove that your body knows what is bad for you: Hold one arm straight out and ask your friend to push your arm down while you resist as hard as you can. Now ask you friend to place a substance (in its container) in a paper sack without your knowing the contents. The substance could be something poisonous if consumed, or a food/medication good for you. Place the sack on your lap, near your free hand or your feet. Repeat the arm exercise. When the substance is poisonous, your arm will give way. If the substance is good for you, you will have extra resistance.

Now try testing yourself. Make a circle with your forefinger and thumb. With the other hand, use your middle finger or forefinger to try and break the circle. Notice the difference when you are holding a can of something poisonous. This is the reaction you will get if you are allergic to something in a container of supplements. Test every supplement before you buy it and remember to test again if you change brands.

3. Eat a balanced diet You will crave more variety of foods as you begin to get well. Vitamin and mineral sources are listed freely in books, stores, etc. I have listed sources for enzymes and amino acids in the back of this book. The need for variety in your diet will be obvious. Look up the food sources for the nutrients that you were low on and add some of those foods to your regular diet.

4. Examine your thinking. Do some soul searching about why you are here on earth and what thoughts or beliefs have caused you unhappiness. **Illness is caused 50% by malnutrition and 50% by wrong thinking.** You may benefit from reading books about self-examination. See the two recommended in the Question and Answer section.

SYMPTOMS OF A THYROID BLOCKAGE

A person with any four or more of the following symptoms will probably have a thyroid blockage **provided blood tests indicate no thyroid abnormality.**

- **Inability to handle extreme air temperatures of either hot or cold.** Earliest childhood memories may be of being cold.

- **Cold skin even when you work up a sweat.**

- Having to force yourself out of bed every day for years. A **distinct feeling that you have less energy than others.**

- **Hair color turns darker** in 40's rather than turning gray or white.

- Indications of **arthritis as a juvenile.**

- **A double chin.** The Universal Force says that no one should have a double chin. This condition always indicates a problem with the thyroid.

- A **craving for dairy food and calcium deposits (lumps)** under the skin. This condition occurs because the parathyroid is not functioning properly. The parathyroid is unable to digest calcium when thyroxin is low.

- Difficulty with **digestion.** Problems can include intestinal gas, constipation, and/or diarrhea.

- **Abnormally large eyes.** If you see a picture of the person in a group, do his or her eyes jump out at you?

- **High and low blood pressure**—It is common for a person with thyroid blockage to experience both at different times in life. Note: When thyroid medication is at the proper level, blood pressure is normal. Every person with high blood pressure has a thyroid problem—either high, low, or blocked.

- **Irregular menstrual cycles/periods** in women. Older women will frequently have had hysterectomies.

- A **vision change** from farsighted or nearsighted to the other. Also **scratchy, dry eyes.**

- **Alkaline body rather than acid.** This results in itchy skin, a tendency for yeast infections, slow healing of scratches and wounds.

- An itch, which when scratched, develops into **something that looks like poison ivy.** May be caused by grease, oil, sap of plants etc. if not washed off immediately. Can take weeks to heal.

- **Inability to tolerate humidity at any temperature.** Person may become very nervous as a result of being in a humid room.

- **Craving for caffeine** such as colas, coffee, and chocolate. This is a craving for energy.

- **Overweight whether overeating or not.** When you lack thyroid, you have slow metabolism but you may also get hungry more often. Heavy people who rarely overeat usually have either low thyroid or blocked thyroid.

- Diagnosed with sleep apnea.

- **Dowager's hump.** Without enough thyroid, the body deposits fat at the base of the neck. Given thyroid, the body slowly utilizes the fat by burning it as energy.

- Heredity—Relatives with low thyroid and/or many of the above symptoms.

What To Do If You Have A Blocked Thyroid

1. Try to find a holistic physician, especially one who might dowse or do intuitive work to conform your suspicions. If not possible, try to find someone who has been dowsing for several years.

2. Go to a health food store and purchase thyroid in about 30 milligram (mg.) strength. (Order, if necessary).

   Note: Whether prescription or over-the-counter, number of milligrams should be the same or as close as possible.

   Also, over-the-counter glandular thyroid is better than non-glandular. Even though there is no thyroxin in over-the-counter, taking it will produce the same effect. Non-glandular thyroid should only be used by persons who get adverse reactions to red meat.

3. Cut four pills in half. Take one half pill or 15 **mg.** of thyroid extract for 8 days.

4. Then take approximately 30 mg. for the next 6 months. If you feel fine at the end of 6 months, this is the dose you should continue taking until your blockage is removed.

5. If you find no relief of symptoms after 6 months, go to 60mg. for the next 10 months.

6. If symptoms persist after 10 months, increase thyroid to 90 mg. for 3 months. After 3 months at 90 mg. either symptoms will subside or you will need to go to

increase the dosage. A higher dosage by only 15 mg. (105mg. total). **Most patients will only need 60 mg. or less.**

If your blood pressure <u>increases</u> (you get heart palpitations) after being on a single dose of thyroid for several months, you have a **resistance.** This means your body is resisting foreign thyroid. Continue taking the thyroid; the resistance will wear off eventually. **Heart palpitations indicate a need for 99mg. of potassium per day. <u>Increase</u> potassium by 1 pill every 9 days until heart palpitations stop. (If you ever get up to 9 (99mg) potassium pills, <u>and heart palpitations continue, increase </u>the thyroid dose again). Continue for 8 days. <u>Decrease</u> potassium by 1 pill every 8 days. Repeat this process until taking only 1 potassium pill. When heart palpitations have stopped, discontinue potassium. You are at the correct level of thyroid for your body when blood pressure remains normal without potassium.**

I feel obligated to warn you that at some point in this process, you may have to go against doctor's orders in an effort to reach a point where you finally feel **well.** If you are going to do this on your own, you should still tell any physician treating you about the medication you are on.

Also, be aware that a low thyroid condition makes zinc unavailable to the body.

7. When you begin to attain more thyroxin in your system, some of your symptoms will begin to reverse themselves. Continue treatment; this indicates the medicine is working.

8. Pray to God—or whatever you believe in—to make the blockage go away.

WHAT IS A THYROID BLOCKAGE?

The average thyroid gland produces about 210 milligrams of thyroxine each day. Most people only use 130 mg./day and the remainder (80mg.) leaves the body in urine. That is how it works in a normal, healthy, body. If you have a blockage, there will be 90 mg. or more of thyroxine in the urine. A person can live with a 10-15% blockage. A blockage of 20% or more will deter some sort of function within the body. The effect depends upon exactly what area is blocked so different people have different symptoms. I have a 60% blockage and about 125mg. of thyroxine are leaving my body daily. My body requires 120mg. of supplemental thyroid medication. I get 40% of my own thyroxin production (210mg. x .40 = 84mg.) **plus 40% of the supplement I take** (120mg. x .40 = 48mg.). Together that is 132 mg.(84mg. + 48mg.)—about what every person uses. NOTE: The per cent of blockage represents the amount of ALL your medications being blocked. If you have a thyroid blockage you may be taking higher than average doses of medicines to obtain the desired effects.

What causes a thyroid blockage?

According to the Universal Force, these blockages are due to injuries experienced in past lives but retained in cell memory. To block the thyroid, the injury had to occur between the chin and the base of the throat. It could have been on the front of the throat, on the side, or even on the back of the neck. I believe that I was hanged in a past lifetime. If you think about where a rope would hit a person being hanged, it is easy to understand it would effect the thyroid area.

Does this blockage show up on any medical tests?

The Universal Force says this blockage would show up on a CAT scan, MRI, and/or ultrasound as abnormal energy in the area of the blockage. The blockage does not appear as a physical or solid substance. The reason it does not indicate low thyroid in blood tests is because the adequate amount of thyroid is in the blood. There simply **is not enough blood**. The per cent of blockage also represents how much less blood is in the body than that of a normal person.

How many people have this problem?

The Universal Force provided these figures:

12% of the world population has hypothyroid—too little thyroxine—which can be cured (see Illnesses). This condition is diagnosed via blood tests, specifically T3, T4, and TSH. Hypothyroid patients have many of the same symptoms as those with a blockage.

15% of the world population has a thyroid blockage like myself. Included in this number is 4% of us who experience a resistance to the medication in addition to the blockage.

A very small number of persons will have both hypothyroid and a thyroid blockage as well.

Mental Illnesses

> Warning: Mental patients on psychotropic drugs must stay on the drugs until cured. Symptoms will get worse as they approach cure because psychotropic drugs have opposite effects on healthy people. If patient's symptoms get worse it means he or she is cured. Stop giving psychotropic medication *and* essential nutrient.

Addiction, Prescription Medications, Colas

Essential: Vitamin B-6
Helpful: L-Alanine, L-arginine, cholin, biotin
Maximum Cure Time: 6 Weeks

Addiction, Narcotics, Street Drugs, Gambling, Kleptomania, Sex, Food

Essential: L-Cysteine
Helpful: Vitamins A, B complex, D, wheat germ
Maximum Cure Time: 9 Months

Alcoholism

Essential: Chromium
Helpful: Vitamins A, B complex, K, spirulina, selenium, alfalfa
Maximum Cure Time: 24 Days

Alzheimer's' Disease *see also* Senile Dementia

Essential: This disease is a result of Blocked Thyroid. *See* **What To Do If You Have A Blocked Thyroid** in front section of book.
Helpful: Acidophilus, alfalfa, astralagus, damiana, ginkgo biloba, Siberian ginseng, rhubarb root, skullcap, slippery elm, uva ursi, watercress
Maximum Cure Time: 10 Months
About 20% of Alzheimer's' patients actually have Senile Dementia and have been misdiagnosed.

Amnesia

Essential: Pancreatine NF
Helpful: L-Cystine, L-glycine, L-histidine, L-proline, L-serine, L-taurine, L-threonine, L-tryosine
Maximum Cure Time: 3 Months

Anorexia

Essential: Vitamin K
Helpful: Amylase, bioflavonoids, evening primrose oil, yarrow
Maximum Cure Time: 4 Weeks

Attention Deficit Disorder *see* Hyperactivity
Autism

Essential: L-Aspartic acid
Helpful: Germanium, cellulose, chlorella, gums/mucilages, green magma, octacosanol, spirulina, suma, uva ursi, cascara sagrada
Maximum Cure Time: 4 Weeks

Battered Wife Syndrome

Essential: Zinc
Helpful: Vitamins B complex, B-3, PABA, all enzymes, L-valine, L-ornithine, octacosanol
Maximum Cure Time: 8 Weeks Also cures Batterer

Bi-Polar *see* Manic-Depression
Body Dysmorphie Disorder (BOD)

Essential: DL-Phenylalaine
Helpful: Germanium, iodine, iron, manganese, lipase, amylase, rutin, catalase, protase, L-hisitidine, gums/mucilages, wheat germ, acidophilus, chlorella, comfrey root, skullcap, thyme, white oak bark
Maximum Cure Time: 4 Months

Bulimia

Essential: Germanium
Helpful: Vitamin B-12, PABA, vanadium, zinc
Maximum Cure Time: 2 Months

Depression—Includes Hoarding—Does NOT Include Post Partum

Essential: Chymotrypsin
Helpful: Boron, L-ornithine, L-phenylalaine, L-lysine
Maximum Cure Time: 6 Months
In the U.S., 70% of depression is caused by the person living and/or working in a building with metal siding. To remedy an existing building with metal siding, encircle the building with house wiring of number 10 or 12 weight or use two strands of the same weight or use a single strand of number 8 copper wire. Leave a gap of 12-48 inches between the two ends. Twist the ends tightly together. Tack or staple the ends on a piece of wood so they are exactly even with each other. This will create a magnetic force. You can bury the entire wire when complete. You must encircle the building with one continuous piece of wire—twisting pieces together will not work.

Fetal Alcohol Syndrome

Essential: Cholin
Helpful: Coenzyme Q10, inositol
Maximum Cure Time: 8 Months

Gender Identity

Essential: Vitamin E
Helpful: Coenzyme Q10, sodium, lipase, amylase, rutin, catalase, acidophilus, aloe vera, bee propolis, desiccated liver, coltsfoot, echinacea, eyebright, feverfew, gotu kola, hawthorn berries, hops, horehound, huckleberries, milkweed, yarrow
Maximum Cure Time: 7 Months
This malady usually develops as a result of malnutrition in the mother during pregnancy but can also develop after the child is born. Adults who have had sex changes should not consider this cure.

Hyperactivity/Attention Deficient Disorder

Essential: Magnesium
Helpful: All vitamins, folic acid, inositol, PABA, sulfur, vanadium, calcium, chromium, copper, germanium, iodine, iron, manganese, molybdenum, phosphorus, potassium, green magma, lecithin, octacosanol, spirulina, wheat germ, suma, white oak bark, hops, licorice root, gentian
Maximum Cure Time: 6 Days
This illness is caused by lifestyle. While 40% is caused by sugar, 30% is caused by microwave ovens. When using a microwave oven, one should stand to the side of the operating appliance. Fewer waves come out the side of the oven. Pregnant women and children should be especially careful not to stand in front of a working microwave oven. Also, 20% of this illness is caused by exposure to **heavy** power lines and 10% is due to lack of folic acid.

Lewy Body Disease

Essential: Sulfur
Helpful: Vitamin E, zinc, all enzymes, L-ornithine, green magma, lecithin, coltsfoot, comfrey root
Maximum Cure Time: 8 Months

Manic-Depression/Bi-Polar

Essential: Folic acid
Helpful: L-proline, L-hisitidine
Maximum Cure Time: 7 Months
Avoid eating all red meat, eggs, salt-water seafood, fresh vegetables, and beans.until cured.

Mental Retardation, Mongolism or Down's Syndrome

Essential: Vanadium
Helpful: Vitamins A, B complex, B-2, B-6, B-12, C, biotin, cholin, inositol, PABA, coenzyme Q10, bromelin, papain, trypsin, chymotrypsin, lipase, amylase, catalase, protase, SOD, all amino acids, acidophilus, cellulose, chlorophyll, garlic,

green magma, lecithin, octacosanol, spirulina, alfalfa, astralagus, black cohosh, black walnut, blue cohosh, horehound
Maximum Cure Time: 2 Years

Mental Retardation, Non-Mongoloid

Essential: L-Methionine
Helpful: Vitamin B complex, B-2, B-3, B-6, B-12, folic acid, all enzymes, brewers' yeast, wheat germ mullein, nettle, pumpkin, yellow dock, yerbamate, horehound, huckleberries, juniper berries, kelp, lobelia
Maximum Cure Time: 9 Months

Multiple Personalities

Essential: Chromium
Helpful: Boron, blessed thistle, blue cohosh, cornsilk, gentian
Maximum Cure Time: 6 Months

Neurosis

Essential: Zinc
Helpful: Evening primrose oil, green magma, chaparral, chickweed, dandelion, hops, licorice root, parsley, psyllium, slippery elm, suma, thyme, yucca
Maximum Cure Time: 5 Days

Obsessive-Compulsive Disorder (OCD)

Essential: Iodine
Helpful: Vitamins A, E, K, catalase, copper, iodine, iron, molybdenum, L-carnitine, L-cysteine, L-cystine, lecithin, gotu kola, hops, huckleberries, Irish moss, peppermint, sarsaparilla, uva ursi, yellow dock, yerbamate
Maximum Cure Time: 4 Months

Paranoia

Essential: Vitamin E
Helpful: Vitamins C, F, bioflavonoids, coenzyme Q10, chymotrypsin, protase, catalase, L-alanine, L-arginine, L-aspartic acid, L-citruline, L-cysteine L-cystine, GABA, L-glycine, L-lysine, L-taurine, L-threonine, L-tryosine, gums/mucilages,

green magma, lecithin, acidophilus, barley grass, cellulose, evening primrose oil, astragalus, black cohosh, black walnut, bladderwrack, blue cohosh, calendula, cascara sagrada, chaparral, coltsfoot, comfrey root, gentian, ginseng, hawthorn berries, hops, horsetail, huckleberries, Irish moss, pau d'arco, pumpkin, water-cress
Maximum Cure Time: 3 Months

Pedophilia

Essential: Folic acid
Helpful: Vitamins B-l, B-6, B-l 2, copper, germanium, iron, magnesium, selenium, silicon, sulfur, trypsin, lipase, amylase, rutin, protase, evening primrose oil, garlic, octacosanol, spirulina, wheat germ, bladderwrack, blue vervain, buchu, burdock root, coltsfoot, feverfew, germander, ginger suma, thyme, uva ursi, yellow dock, yucca
Maximum Cure Time: 7 Months

Post-Partum Depression

Essential: Vitamin A
Helpful: Trypsin, all minerals, DL-phenylalaine, acidolphilus, chlorella, evening primrose oil, gums/mucilages, garlic, black cohosh, feverfew, flaxseed, mullein, peppermint, red raspberry.
Maximum Cure Time: 7 Months

Post-Traumatic Stress Disorder (PTSD)

Essential: Coenzyme Q1O
Helpful: Bioflavonoids, wood betony
Maximum Cure Time: 10 Months

Prader Willi Syndrome

Essential: Coenzyme Q1O
Helpful: Sodium, sulfur, vanadium, zinc, L-citruline, L-glutathine, spirulina, calendula, cascara sagrada, hops, horsetail, thyme, uva ursi, wood betony, yucca, yerbamate
Maximum Cure Time: 1 Year

Psychosis

Essential: L-Taurine
Helpful: Catalase, lecithin
Maximum Cure Time: 5 Weeks

Savant

Essential: Copper
Helpful: Rutin, boron, germanium, selenium, silicon, sodium, vanadium, L-alanine, acidophilus, celery seed, chamomile, red clover, rose hips
Maximum Cure Time: 3 Years
Patients with genius or special talents will retain these after cure.

Schizophrenia, Type I

Essential: Zinc
Helpful: Germanium, potassium, selenium, lobelia, milkweed, vitamin E, pumpkin
Maximum Cure Time: 2 Years

Schizophrenia, Type II

Essential: Vitamin K
Helpful: Rutin, SOD
Maximum Cure Time: 3 Years
About 80% of schizophrenics have Type I and develop the disease in their teens or twenties. Patients who have Type II schizophrenia are usually 45 or older before getting the illness.

Senile Dementia

Essential: Vitamin E
Helpful: All enzymes, L-asparagine, L-aspartic acid, L-carnitine, L-citruline, L-cysteine, L-cystine, GABA, L-glutamic acid, L-glutamine, acidophilus, skullcap, suma, valerian, watercress, yucca, flaxseed, ginger, hawthorn berries, horehound, juniper berries, horsetail, gotu kola, ginkgo biloba, Siberian ginseng, damiana, alfalfa, astralagus
Maximum Cure Time: 10 Months

If you are not certain whether your loved one has Alzheimer's disease (blocked thyroid) or senile dementia, give the patient 1000 IU of vitamin E for a month. If no improvement after one month, it is Alzheimer's.

Smoking Dependency

Essential: Vitamin D
Helpful: Vitamin K, manganese, phosphorus, selenium, all amino acids, spirulina, aloe vera, parsley, ginkgo biloba
Maximum Cure Time: 6 Weeks

Sociopath

Essential: PancreatinNF
Helpful: All vitamins, all amino acids, molybdenum, manganese, selenium, silicon, desiccated liver, garlic, spirulina, chaparral, chickweed, ginger, hops, horehound, horsetail, Irish moss, lobelia, milkweed, red clover, slippery elm, suma, valerian, white oak back, yarrow, yellow dock, yerbamate
Maximum Cure Time: 7 Weeks
Patient will have a conscience when cured. Malnutrition prevents them from connecting with it. *A psychopath* has no conscience and cannot be cured.

Stuttering

Essential: L-Threonine
Helpful: Vitamins A, C, E, K, sodium, vanadium, L-isoleucine, L-leucine, L-methionine, L-ornithine, L-phenylalaine, DL-phenylalaine, L-tryosine, aloe vera, barley grass, bee pollen/honey, brewers' yeast, alfalfa, catnip, celery seed, chamomile, comfrey root, cornsilk, fenugreek, hops, horehound, horsetail, huckleberries, juniper berries, lobelia, milk thistle, pumpkin, sarsaparilla, psyllium, suma, thyme, watercress, yucca
Maximum Cure Time: 2 Weeks

Tourette's Syndrome

Essential: Selenium
Helpful: Copper, sodium, octacosanol, eyebright, uva ursi, yerbamate
Maximum Cure Time: 7 Months

Physical Illnesses

Acne

Essential: Vitamin B-6
Helpful: L-Citraline, L-cystine, bee pollen/honey, bee propolis, brewers' yeast, evening primrose oil, spirulina, yarrow, chamomile, echinacea
Maximum Cure Time: 2 Weeks

Adrenal Disorders

Essential: Iodine
Helpful: Lipase, protase, amylase, Vitamins C, D, E, chlorella, pennyroyal
Maximum Cure Time: 5 Months

AID see HIV-AIDS
Albino (Lack of Pigmentation)

Essential: Germander
Helpful: Wood betony
Maximum Cure Time: 5 Years
If blind from this disease, vision should return with this remedy.

Allergies

Reactions to corn, wheat, soy, and tree nuts are due to cell memory from a prior lifetime.
The following reactions result from malnutrition.
Maximum Cure Time for each is 10 weeks.

Eggs: Boron

Peanuts: Bromelin

Shellfish: L-Valine

Yeast: Vitamin K

Dairy: Trypsin

Gluten: L-Lysine

Sulfur: SOD

Penicillin: SOD

ALS *see* Lou Gerhig's Disease
Aneurism, Brain

Essential: Vitamin F
Helpful: Pancreatine NF, bromelin, lipase, catalase, protase, cellulose, evening primrose oil, comfrey root, Echinacea, fennel, flaxseed, germander
Maximum Cure Time: 2 Weeks

Aneurism, Except Brain

Essential: Vitamin F
Helpful: Silicon, sodium, vanadium, rutin, L-ornithine, evening primrose oil, blue cohosh, blue vervain, suma, thyme, watercress, wood betony, yarrow, yerbamate
Maximum Cure Time: 7 Weeks

Angina Pectoris *also* Myocardial Infarction

Essential: Pancreatine NF
Helpful: Zinc, rutin, bee propolis, brewers yeast, chlorella, garlic octocosanol, spriulina, wheat germ, buchu, cascara sagrada, chaparral, cornsilk, dandelion
Maximum Cure Time: 1 Month

Anthrax

Essential: Vitamin K
Helpful: Garlic, alfalfa, sarsaparilla, milkweed
Maximum Cure Time: 3 Months

Appetite, Excessive

Essential: L-Cysteine
Helpful: Vitamin C, L-asparagine, GABA, cascara sagrada, milkweed, flaxseed, goldenseal
Maximum Cure Time: 5 Days

Appetite, Poor

Essential: Bromelin
Helpful: Papain
Maximum Cure Time: 4 Days

Arteriosclerosis (Hardening of the Arteries)

Essential: Phosphorus
Helpful: Potassium, Vitamin D, pancreatine NF, bromelin, trypsin, wheat germ, capsicum
Maximum Cure Time: 2 Years

Arthritis, Osteoarthritis

Essential: Copper
Helpful: Boron, bee pollen/honey, evening primrose oil, capsicum, hawthorn berries, huckleberries, juniper berries
Maximum Cure Time: 3 Years

Arthritis, Rheumatoid

Essential: Vitamin D
Helpful: Vitamins A, C, E, K, biotin, folic acid, inositol, pancreatin NF, bromelin, papain, trypsin, chymotrypsin, rutin, protase, barley grass, bee pollen/honey, bee propolis, evening primrose oil, gums/mucilages, alfalfa, sarsaparilla
Maximum Cure Time: 8 Years

Asbestos Poisoning

Essential: L-Leucine
Helpful: L-Alanine, damiana, juniper berries
Maximum Cure Time: 2 Years

Asthma

Essential: L-Glycine
Helpful: Vitamin C, wheat germ, Irish moss
Maximum Cure Time: 4 Months

Athlete's Foot

Essential: L-Cysteine
Helpful: Chlorophyll, slippery elm, bladder wrack
Maximum Cure Time: 3 Weeks

Bedsores

Essential: Yerbamate—apply Externally to sores, do NOT take internally.
Helpful: Trypsin, amylase
Maximum Cure Time: 4 days

Bedwetting

Essential: Vitamin B-2
Maximum Cure Time: 2 Weeks

Bee Sting

Essential: Amylase
Maximum Cure Time: 2 Minutes

Beriberi

Essential: Vitamin B Complex
Helpful: Magnesium, bee pollen/honey, desiccated liver, yerbamate
Maximum Cure Time: 5 Weeks

Bladder Control

Essential: Vitamin A
Helpful: Vitamins D, E, Coenzyme Q10, red clover, rose hops
Maximum Cure Time: 14 Days

Boils

Essential: Rutin
Helpful: Garlic
Maximum Cure Time: 7 Days

Brain Injury

Essential: L-Glycine
Helpful: Vitamins B-1, B-2, B-3, B-5, B-6, calcium, chromium, iodine, phenyla-laine, wheat germ, brewers' yeast, pumpkin
Maximum Cure Time: 3 Months

Bruising

Essential: Vitamin A
Helpful: Green Magma, evening primrose oil, catnip, watercress, yarrow
Maximum Cure Time: 2 Weeks

Bruxism

Essential: Iodine
Helpful: All amino acids, aloe vera, octacosanol, wheat germ, Echinacea, haw-thorn berries
Maximum Cure Time: 2 Weeks

Bubonic Plague

Essential: Silicon
Helpful: Vitamins B-1, B-2, B-5, B-6, B-12, E, F, K, bioflavonoids, folic acid, inositol, PABA, coenzyme Q10, all amino acids, lecithin, calendula, catnip, celery seed, coltsfoot, corn silk, damiana, dandelion, germander, ginger, gotu kola, grindelia, hawthorn berries, hops, horehound, horsetail, huckleberries, Irish moss, juniper berries, licorice root, lobelia, milk thistle, milkweed
Maximum Cure Time: 2 Months

Burns

Essential: Zinc-ORALLY ONLY
        Aloe vera—EXTERNALLY ONLY
Helpful: Silicon, rutin, brewers yeast, catnip, coltsfoot
Maximum Cure Time: 2 Months

Bursitis

Essential: L-Lysine
Helpful: Sulfur, L-leucine, L-cysteine, L-serine, L-tryosine, catnip, suma
Maximum Cure Time: 1 Month

Calluses

Essential: PABA
Helpful: Vitamins A, B-2, B-3, B-5, B-6, D, E, K, bioflavonoids, coenzyme Q10, inositol, amylase, rutin, SOD, protase, L-glycine, L-histidine, L-phenylalaine, DL-phenylalaine, L-serine, L-taurine, L-tryptophan, L-ornithine, green magma, barley grass, cellulose, alfalfa, barberry, blue cohosh, buchu, butcher's broom, fenugreek, gotu kola, hops, uva ursi, valerian, yellow dock
Maximum Cure Time: 10 Days

Cancer, Bladder and Kidney

Essential: Trypsin
Helpful: Vitamins B-5, D, bioflavonoids, coenzyme Q10, pancreatine NF, bromeline, lipase
Maximum Cure Time: 5 Months

Cancer, Bone

Essential: L-Leucine
Helpful: Vitamin B-2, manganese, iron, iodine, chromium
Maximum Cure Time: 2 Years

Cancer, Brain

Essential: L-Ornithine
Helpful: Vitamins B-2, B-3, D, biotin, folic acid, cholin, L-cysteine, L-cystine, L-citruline, green magma, fenugreek, feverfew, flaxseed, goldenseal, gingko biloba, licorice root
Maximum Cure Time: 2 Years

Cancer, Breast—Type I

Occurs in women aged 30 or older. 80% of Breast Cancer is Type I
Essential: Bioflavonoids
Helpful: Vitamins E, F, amylase
Maximum Cure Time: 2 Years

Cancer, Breast—Type II

Occurs in males only. Accounts for 15% of Breast Cancer cases.
Essential: L-Leucine
Helpful: L-Taurine, L-tyrosine, chromium, amylase
Maximum Cure Time: 2 Years

Cancer, Breast—Type III

Occurs in women aged 29 and under. Accounts for 5% of Breast Cancer cases.
Essential: Vitamin B-6
Helpful: Vitamin B Complex, vitamin E, licorice root
Maximum Cure Time: 2 Year

Cancer, Cervical

Essential: Zinc
Helpful: Bladderwrack, blue vera vain, buchu, butcher's broom, catnip, colts-foot, cornsilk, Irish moss
Maximum Cure Time: 7 Months

Cancer, Colon

Essential: L-Carnitine
Helpful: Calcium, manganese, phosphorus, sulfur, SOD, octacosanol, bee propolis, cellulose, chlorella, chlorophyll, barberry, black walnut
Maximum Cure Time: 1 Year

Cancer, Hodgkin's Disease *see* Cancer, Brain
Cancer, Leukemia

Essential: L-Cysteine

Helpful: Iodine, phosphorus, sodium, L-asparagine, L-carnitine, L-citruline, L-glutamine, L-threonine brewers' yeast, chlorophyll, garlic, green magma, bladder wrack, cascara sagrada, flaxseed, hops, horehound, huckleberries, Irish moss, licorice root
Maximum Cure Time: 10 Months

Cancer, Lung

Essential: GABA
Helpful: L-Asparagine, L-aspartic acid, L-cysteine, trypsin, garlic, green magma, octocosanol, butcher's broom, goldenseal
Maximum Cure Time: 4 Months

Cancer, Lymphoma

Essential: L-Isoleucine
Helpful: Vitamin B-2, biotin, folic acid, inositol, PABA, copper, iodine, manganese, L-cystine, L-isoleucine, L-ornithine, DL-phenylalaine, proline, aloe vera, bee pollen/honey, bee propolis, evening primrose oil, black walnut, bladder wrack, blue vervain, capsicum, cascara sagrada, chaparral, damiana, Irish moss, milk thistle, milkweed, red clover, red raspberry, white oak bark, yellow dock, watercress, thyme, wheat germ
Maximum Cure Time: 1 Year

Cancer, Multiple Myeloma

Essential: Catalase
Helpful: Vitamins C, K, bioflavonoids, PABA, potassium, pancreatine NF, papain, trypsin, rutin, protase, SOD, L-Lysine
Maximum Cure Time: 7 Months

Cancer, Mouth

Essential: L-Asparagine
Helpful: Vitamin C, silicon, vanadium
Maximum Cure Time: 5 Months

Cancer, Ovarian and Uterine

Essential: Folic acid
Helpful: Cholin, inositol, catalase, all amino acids, chlorophyll, garlic, uva ursi, watercress, hawthorn berries
Maximum Cure Time: 8 Months

Cancer, Pancreatic

Essential: Bromelin
Helpful: Coenzyme Q10, L-glutamine, L-glutathione, pancreatine, trypsine, chymotrypsin, protase, amylase, rutin, SOD, catalase, octacosanol, gums/mucilages, wheat germ, alfalfa, capsicum, cascara sagrada, hawthorn berries, hops, milk thistle, juniper berries, huckle berries, Irish moss
Maximum Cure Time: 2 Years

Cancer, Prostate

Essential: Germanium
Helpful: PABA, vitamin B complex, chamomile, chaparral, comfrey root, ginger, horehound, Irish moss, juniper berries, milk thistle, milkweed, uva ursi
Maximum Cure Time: 3 Years

Cancer, Skin

Essential: Vitamin D
Helpful: Vitamin B-2, biotin, L-asparagine, L-carnitine, potassium, chlorella
Maximum Cure Time: 2 Years
Note: Use of sun screen **increases** your chances of getting skin cancer because you need Vitamin D on a daily basis. Adults need to be exposed to the sun about 60 minutes a day, children about 40 minutes.

Cancer, Stomach

Essential: Vitamin B Complex
Helpful: Wheat germ, lecithin, damiana, evening primrose oil
Maximum Cure Time: 8 Weeks

Cancer, Testicular

Essential: Biotin
Helpful: Boron, Siberian ginseng
Maximum Cure Time: 2 Months

Cancer, Throat

Essential: Vitamin D
Helpful: Coenzyme Q10, iodine
Maximum Cure Time: 3 Months

Cancer, Thyroid

Essential: L-Serine
Helpful: Coenzyme Q10, iodine, tryptophan, tyrosine, barley grass, spriulina, nettle, red raspberry, sarsaparilla, alfalfa, red clover
Maximum Cure Time: 2 Months

Candidiasis

Essential: Vitamin K
Helpful: Acidophilus, bee pollen/honey, bee propolis
Maximum Cure Time: 9 Weeks

Canker Sores

Essential: Zinc-APPLIED EXTERNALLY ONLY
Helpful: Vitamin E, bioflavonoids, L-isoleucine, L-ornithine, L-phenylalaine, DL-phenylalaine, L-serine, L-taurine, L-threonine, L-tryptophan, L-tryosine, cellulose, catnip, grindelia
Maximum Cure Time: 2 Hours

Carpal Tunnel Syndrome

Essential: PABA
Helpful: Vitamins B-3, B-5, folic acid, inositol, trypsin, L-isoleucine, DL-phenylalaine, L-proline, L-serine, L-taurine, L-tryptophan, germander, Siberian ginseng, goldenseal, psyllium

Maximum Cure Time: 9 Weeks

Cerebral Palsy

Essential: Vitamin B-3
Helpful: Vitamin B Complex, Vitamins B-l, B-2, C, D, E, F, K, bioflavonoids, coenzyme Q10, biotin, cholin, folic acid, inositol, potassium, molybdenum, chlorella, disiccated liver
Maximum Cure Time: 8 Months

Chafing

Essential: Coenzyme Q10
Helpful: Vitamins A, C, rose hips
Maximum Cure time: 2 Days

Chapped Hands

Essential: L-Carnitine
Helpful: Vitamins B-2, B-3, bioflavonoids, folic acid, cornsilk, dandelion, hawthorn berries, hops, huckleberries, yellow dock, yarrow, bee propolis, brewers yeast Zinc-EXTERNALLY ONLY
Maximum Cure Time: 1 Hour

Chicken Pox

Essential: L-Lysine
Helpful: Cellulose, octacosanol
Maximum Cure Time: 7 Days

Chlamydia

Essential: Vitamin B-5
Helpful: Biotin, phosphorus, lecithin
Maximum Cure Time: 7 Days

Cholera

Essential: Rutin

Helpful: Molybdenum, sulfur, L-lysine, L-valine, L-methionine, L-ornithine, DL-phenylalaine, L-phenylalaine, L-proline
Maximum Cure Time: 2 Months

Chronic Fatigue Syndrome

This illness is the result of Blocked Thyroid *See* **What to do If You Have a Blocked Thyroid** in front section of book.

Cirrhosis of the Liver

Essential: L-Isoleucine
Helpful: Copper, iodine
Maximum Cure Time: 4 Years

Circulatory Problems

Essential: Bromelin
Helpful: L-Histidine, DL-phenylalaine, L-asparagines, L-citruline, octacosanol, catnip, pennyroyal, blue cohosh
Maximum Cure Time: 7 Months

CJD *see* Mad Cow Disease
Colitis

Essential: Folic acid
Helpful: Biotin, cholin, eornsilk, milk thistle, coenzyme Q10
Maximum Cure Time: 5 Weeks

Common Cold and Viral Infections, *see also* Flu, and RSV

Essential: Vitamin B-12
Helpful: Vitamin B-2, calcium, horehound
Maximum Cure Time: 1 Day

Cold Sores

Essential: Vitamin B Complex
Helpful: Calcium
        Apply zinc ointment
Maximum Cure Time: 2 Weeks

Congestive Heart Failure *see* Heart

Constipation

Essential: L-Tryptophan
Helpful: Vitamin K, coenzyme Q10, papain, protase, calcium, magnesium, manganese, molybdenum, L-lysine, L-phenylalaine, L-proline, cellulose, green magma, alfalfa, cornsilk, flaxseed, hawthorn berries, hops, horehound, huckleberries, juniper berries, milk thistle, parsley, peppermint, psyllium, pumpkin
Maximum Cure Time: 1 Hour

Copper Toxicity

Essential: Pancreatine NF
Helpful: Lipase, papain, octacosanol
Maximum Cure Time: 5 Months

Corns

Essential: Iodine—internally only
Helpful: L-Lysine, L-glycine, germander, ginger, kelp, lobelia
Maximum Cure Time: 2 Weeks

Crohn's Disease

Essential: Trypsin
Helpful: L-Ornithine
Maximum Cure Time: 4 Months

Croup

Essential: Phosphorus
Helpful: SOD, boron, Vitamins B-2, B-6, folic acid, garlic, green magma

Maximum Cure Time: 4 Days

Cystic Fibrosis

Essential: L-Asparagine
Helpful: Grindelia
Maximum Cure Time: 7 Months

Dandruff

Essential: L-Alanine
Helpful: Chapparral, butcher's broom, cornsilk, milkweed, parsley, yerbamate— internally
        Nettle-EXTERNALLY ONLY
Maximum Cure Time: 2 Weeks

Deafness

Essential: Vitamin F
Helpful: Papain, lipase, amylase, protase, catalase, vanadium, all amino acids, evening primrose oil, barley grass, wheat germ, catnip
Maximum Cure Time: 8 Months

Dental Cavities

Essential: Vitamin K
Helpful: Vitamins B-1, B-2, B-12, cholin, folic acid, inositol, amylase, rutin, catalase, SOD, protase, chromium, molybdenum, sodium, sulfur, zinc, all amino acids, green magma, spiralina, wheat germ, acidophilus, aloe vera, barley grass, bee pollen/honey, bee propolis, brewers yeast, cellulose, chlorella, chlorophyll, desiccated liver, evening primrose oil, alfalfa, astralagus, barberry, blessed thistle, chamomile, coltsfoot, comfrey root, damiana, black walnut, fenugreek, feverfew, gentian, germander, ginger, ginkgo biloba, kelp, lobelia, rhubarb root
Maximum Cure Time: 5 Months

Dermatitis and Eczema

Essential: L-Histidine
Helpful: PABA, butcher's broom, cornsilk, yerbamate

Nettle-EXTERNALLY ONLY
Maximum Cure Time: 6 Months

Diabetes

Essential: L-Valine
Helpful: Gotu kola, blessed thistle
Maximum Cure Time: 2 Months
Most diabetics will need L-valine and both herbs. Take until blood sugar is normal.

Diarrhea

Essential: Vanadium
Helpful: Silicon, sulfur, bioflavonoids, zinc
Maximum Cure Time: 4 Hours

Diphtheria

Essential: Folic acid
Helpful: Vitamins C, E, coenzyme Q10, inositol, PABA, sulfur, zinc, all enzymes, L-threonine, L-tryptophan, L-serine, lecithin octacosanol, spirulina, wheat germ, barley grass, brewers yeast, cellulose, desiccated liver, dandelion, hawthorn berries, horehound, huckleberries, juniper berries, kelp, licorice root, lobelia
Maximum Cure Time: 2 Months

Diverticulitis

Essential: L-Valine
Helpful: L-Arginine, green magma, octacosanol, molybdenum
Maximum Cure Time: 7 Months

Dry Skin

Essential: Coenzyme Q10
Helpful: Cholin, inositol, sodium, papain, skullcap, valerian, flax oil—internally
Maximum Cure Time: 1 Day

Dysentery

Essential: L-Isoleucine
Helpful: Molybdenum, vanadium, L-histidine, L-leucine, L-lysine, L-methionine, L-ornithine, L-phenylalaine, DL-phenylalaine, brewers' yeast, chlorella, spirulina, milk thistle
Maximum Cure Time: 7 Days

Dyslexia

Essential: L-Glycine
Helpful: Butcher's broom, dong quai
Maximum Cure Time: 6 Months

Ear Ache

Essential: Vitamin B Complex
Helpful: Vitamins A, C, D E K, bioflavonoids, all B vitamins, L-carnitine, L-cit-ruline, L-cystine, L-cysteine, GABA, L-glutamic acid, L-glutamine, L-glutathine, L-valine, L-glycine, L-histidine, L-isoleucine, L-leucine, L-lysine, L-methionine, L-ornithine, L-phenylalaine, L-serine, L-taurine, L-threonine, L-tryptophan, L-tryosine, chlorophyll, pau d'arco, calendula, chamomile, chickweed, coltsfoot
Maximum Cure Time: 1 Hour

Ear Infection

Essential: Vitamin B-5
Helpful: Lipase, L-histidine, L-ornithine, L-tryptophan
Maximum Cure Time: 2 Days

Ear Wax

Essential: L-Histidine
Helpful: Vitamin D, L-glycine, L-tryptophan, green magma
Maximum Cure Time: 6 Days

Ears, Ringing *see* Meneire's Syndrome
Ebola, also Marburg

Essential: Vitamin F
Helpful: Evening primrose oil, flax oil, olive oil, safflower oil, fish oil
Maximum Cure Time: 5 Months

E-Coli

Essential: Trypsin
Helpful: Vitamin F, L-valine, L-phenylalaine, L-taurine, calendula, coltsfoot, damiana, evening primrose oil
Maximum Cure Time: 4 Hours

Eczema *see* Dermatitis
Edema

Essential: Vitamin A
Helpful: Vitamin K, B-6, B-12, cholin, folic acid, coenzyme Q10, pancreatine NF, papain, trypsin, chymotrypsin, lipase, amuylase, catalase, protase, all minerals, parsley
Maximum Cure Time: 3 Weeks

Emphysema

Essential: Rutin
Helpful: Vitamins A, C, D, E, K, bioflavonoids, coenzyme Q10, L-glycine, L-isoleucine, L-lysine, L-methionine, L-phenylalaine, L-serine, papain, wheat germ, milkweed
Maximum Cure Time: 6 Weeks

Endometriosis

Essential: Selenium
Helpful: GABA, spriulina
Maximum Cure Time: 6 Weeks
Eliminate corn, citrus fruits, eggs, bananas, rye, and wheat from the diet until cured.

Epilepsy

Essential: Folic acid
Helpful: Vitamin B-5, PABA, gums/mucilages, damiana, burdock root
Maximum Cure Time: 2 Years

Epstein Barr Virus

Essential: Potassium
Helpful: All vitamins, silicon, lipase, green magma, watercress, horsetail, colts-foot, dandelion
Maximum Cure Time: 2 Years

Eyes, Bitot's Spots

Essential: Folic acid
Helpful: Biotin, cholin, L-cysteine, GABA, L-glutamine, L-glutathine, L-valine, cornsilk, celery seed
Maximum Cure Time: 5 Weeks

Eyes, Blindness

Essential: Coenzyme Q10
Helpful: Selenium, L-glutamine, L-glutathine, L-valine, L-phenylalaine, eye-bright, coltsfoot, sarsparilla
Maximum Cure Time: 8 Years
For blindness due to injury, diabetes, and other causes.

Eyes, Blurred Vision

Essential: SOD
Helpful: L-Cysteine, catalase, acidophilus
Maximum Cure Time: 3 Hours

Eyes, Cataracts

Essential: Iron
Helpful: Inositol, chromium, iodine, silicon, sulfur, L-methionine, L-tryptophan
Maximum Cure Time: 2 Years

Person is sleeping too much. Person should also avoid eating cheese, meat, and seafood.

Eyes, Color Blindness

Essential: Coenzyme Q1O
Helpful: Vitamin B complex, vitamins D, E, bioflavonoids, spirulina
Maximum Cure Time: 4 Years

Eyes, Farsightedness (Hyperopia)

Essential: L-Arginine
Helpful: L-Lysine, PABA, inosistol, gentian, watercress
Maximum Cure Time: *2* Years

Eyes, "Floaters"

Essential: Folic acid
Helpful: Inositol, boron, calcium, chromium, protase
Maximum Cure Time: 7 Days

Eyes, Glaucoma

Essential: Catalase
Helpful: Evening primrose oil, lecithin, octacosanol, uva ursi, watercress, celery seed, ginkgo biloba
Maximum Cure Time: 4 Months

Eyes, Itchy

Essential: Vitamin C
Helpful: Vitamin B complex, vitamin D, calcium, copper, germanium, iodine, magnesium, manganese, molybdenum, corn silk
Maximum Cure Time: 2 Days

Eyes, Macular Degeneration

Essential: L-Isoleucine
Helpful: L-Leucine, Vitamins A, K, alfalfa

Maximum Cure Time: 5 Months

Eyes, Nearsightness

Essential: L-Ornithine
Helpful: L-Histidine, L-isoleucine, folic acid. Vitamin B-3
Maximum Cure Time: 9 Weeks

Eyes, Night Blindness

Essential: L-Threonine
Maximum Cure Time: 2 Hours

Eyes, Pain Behind Eye

Essential: L-Phenylalaine
Helpful: Vitamin B complex, bioflavonoids, selenium, sodium, L-arginine, L-asparagine, L-histidine, L-isoleucine, L-methionine, GABA, AOX/PLX*
Maximum Cure Time: 6 Days
*Brand name product available in some health food stores.

Eyes, Photophobia (Light Sensitivity)

Essential: Lipase
Helpful: Amylase, bromelin, pancreatin NF, lecithin, ginkgo biloba
Maximum Cure Time: 8 Months

Eyes, Retinal Edema, Retinal Vascular Leakage, Microaneurisms

Essential: Vitamin B-3
Helpful: Vitamins C, E, B-5, PABA, L-glycine, L-isoleucine, L-leucine, L-lysine, L-phenylalaine, L-cystine, L-cystine, L-aspartic acid, L-glutathine, L-valine, bromelin, papain, protase, chymotrypsin, lipase, skullcap, gentian
Maximum Cure Time: 2 Hours

Eyes, Retinitis Pigmatosis

Essential: Vitamin K

Helpful: Chromium, copper, magnesium, molybdenum, phosphorus, potassium, selenium, silicon, papain, rutin, SOD, alfalfa, hawthorn berries, hops, horsetail, huckleberries, juniper berries, lobelia, pau d'arco, pennyroyal, red clover, red raspberry, rhubarb root, thyme, watercress, yellow dock, yerbamate
Maximum Cure Time: 5 Years

Eyes, Styes

Essential: Vitamin B complex
Helpful: Vitamin D, coenzyme Q10, sulfur, zinc, calcium, manganese, molybdenum, selenium, L-asparagine, L-aspartic acid, L-cystine, L-glutamic acid, L-glutamine, L-glutathine, L-valine, L-serine, L-ornithine, L-methionine, L-isoleucine, L-glycine, gums/mucilages
Maximum Cure Time: 2 Days

Eyes, Thinning of Eyelashes

Essential: Vitamin E
Helpful: Vitamins B-3, B-5, B-12, bioflavonoids, cholin, folic acid, rutin, lipase, ehymotrypsin, trypsin, gotu kola, huckleberries
Maximum Cure Time: 2 Years

Eyes, Ulcerated Eye and Ulcerated Eyelids

Essential: Vitamin B-5
Helpful: Vitamins C, D, E, B-3, coenzyme Q10, selenium, calcium, chromium, wheat germ
Maximum Cure Time: 1 Week

Eyes, Xeropthalmia

Essential: Catalase
Helpful: Vitamins B-1, B-2, B-5, biotin, choline, folic acid, inositol, PABA, zinc, vanadium, sodium, silicon, boron, calcium, copper, chromium, iodine, iron, magnesium, molybdenum, potassium, pancreatine NF, bromelin, papain, tryosine, protase, chymotrypsin, lipase, rutin, SOD, L-histidine, L-lysine, L-ornithine, L-phenylalaine, DL-phenylalaine, GABA, L-proline, L-taurine, L-tyrosine, L-alanine, L-asparagine, L-aspartic acid, L-carnitine, L-cysteine, L-glutamic acid, L-glutamine, L-glutathine, L-valine, parsley, cornsilk

Maximum Cure Time: 6 Months

Eczema *see* Dermatitis
Fatal Familial Insomnia

Essential: Vitamin E
Helpful: Vitamin B Complex, cholin, PABA, L-isoleucine, L-leucine, L-proline, gums/mucilages, garlic, octacosanol, echinacea
Maximum Cure Time: 1 Year

Fever

Essential: Vitamin C
Helpful: Vitamins A, B complex, D, E, K, coenzyme Q10, selenium, zinc, boron, calcium, copper, germanium, iodine, iron, magnesium, manganese, phosphorus, potassium, all amino acids, rose hips, slippery elm, watercress
Maximum Cure Time: 6 Hours

Fibrocystic Disease of the Breast

Essential: L-Histidine
Helpful: Vitamin B-2, biotin, folic acid, gums/mucilages, mullein, peppermint
Maximum Cure Time: 1 Year

Fibroids

Essential: L-Tryptophan
Helpful: L-Histidine, spriulina, barley grass, chlorella, evening primrose oil, hops, black cohosh, black walnut, blue vervain, chickweed
Maximum Cure Time: 6 Months

Fissures and Cracked Skin *see* Chapped Hands and Lips
Flim in Throat

Essential: Bioflavonoids
Helpful: Zinc, L-ornithine, DL-phenylalaine, L-proline, L-serine, acidophilus, bee pollen/honey, bee propolis, brewers' yeast, cellulose, chlorophyll, evening

primrose oil, garlic, spirulina, alfalfa, black walnut, chamomile, chickweed, comfrey root, dong quai, echinacea, fennel, fenugreek, feverfew, flaxseed, gentian, germander, goldenseal, gotu kola, grindelia, hawthorn berries, hops, horehound, horsetail, huckleberries, Irish moss, juniper berries, kelp, licorice root, lobelia, milkweed, pennyroyal, red clover, red raspberry, rhubarb root, rose hips, sarsaparilla, pumpkin, suma, valerian, wood betony, yellow dock, yerbamate, yucca
Maximum Cure Time: 1 Hour

Flu/Influenza *see also* Cold

Essential: Rutin
Helpful: Chromium, zinc, L-valine, L-leucine, L-ornithine
Maximum Cure Time: 24 Hours
"An apple a day keeps the doctor away" is a true saying. Rutin is found in apples as well as other foods. If you have a cold, Vitamin B-12 will cure it within 24 hours. If it is still with you after that, you probably have the flu. When in doubt, take both rutin and Vitamin B-12. (Note: Some viruses are neither colds nor flu.)

Flu, Stomach

Essential: Vitamin B complex
Helpful: Vitamins C, K, all minerals except sodium
Maximum Cure Time: 2 Hours

Food Poisoning

Essential: Calcium
Helpful: Vitamin B-6, folic acid, biotin, chromium, iron, magnesium, manganese, potassium, L-histidine, L-leucine, L-lysine, L-methionine, L-ornithine, DL-phenylalaine, L-tryptophan, spriulina, blue cohosh, chaparral, chickweed, comfrey root, alfalfa
Maximum Cure Time: 90 Minutes
Consuming dairy products does not provide enough calcium. Take calcium tablets or pills.

Foot Odors

Essential: Bromelin

Helpful: Iron, germanium, phosphorus, silicon, sodium, sulfur, L-cystine, GABA, L-valine, L-proline, L-glutamic acid, L-glutamine, L-glutathine, tryptophan, psyIlium, chamomile, damiana, iron
Maximum Cure Time: 2 Days

Fractures

Essential: L-Citruline
Helpful: Vitamins B complex, C, D, E, bioflavonoids, L-asparagine, L-carnitine, L-Glutamic acid, brewers yeast
Maximum Cure Time: 4 Weeks

Frigidity

Essential: Vitamin K
Helpful: Vitamin C, bioflavonoids, lipase, rutin, SOD, selenium, silicon, sulfur, L-histidine, L-methionine, L-phenylalaine, L-proline, L-taurine, L-threonine, L-tryptophan, L-alanine, L-citruline, L-cysteine, L-glutamic acid, L-glutamine, alfalfa, Irish moss
Maximum Cure Time: 2 Weeks

Frostbite

Essential: Sulfur
Helpful: Coenzyme Q10, cholin, sodium, acidophilus, bee propolis, catnip, chamomile, yerbamate
Maximum Cure Time: 2 Hours

Gallbladder Disorders

Essential: Molybdenum
Helpful: Boron, chromium, germanium, iodine, magnesium, watercress
Maximum Cure Time: 2 Months

Gangrene

Essential: L-Isoleucine
Helpful: L-Glycine, L-tryosine, phosphorus, papain, Vitamins A, B-l, B-3, B-5, B-6, B-12, folic acid, capsicum, coltsfoot, Echinacea, gentian, horehound

Maximum Cure Time: 9 Days

Goiter

Essential: L-Methionine
Helpful: Gums/mucilages, blue cohosh, burdockroot
Maximum Cure Time: 2 Days

Gout

Essential: Pancreatine NF
Helpful: Vitamins A, C, E, B-l, B-2, B-5, B-6, B-l2, cholin, inositol, bioflavonoids, protase, L-alanine, L-asparagines, L-aspartic acid, L-citruline, L-cysteine, L-cystine, L-glutathine, L-histidine, L-isoleucine, L-leucine, L-ornithine, L-phenylalaine, gums/mucilages, octacosanol
Maximum Cure Time: 7 Months

Hair Loss

Essential: L-Leucine
Helpful: Vitamins A, C, D, K, coenzyme Q10, L-isoleucine, L-methionine, L-ornithine, GABA, L-taurine, L-tryosine, celery seed, bee propolis
Maximum Cure Time: 3 Weeks Stops loss and adds new growth.

Halitosis

Essential: Vitamin B-l
Helpful: Vitamin B-3, B-6, biotin, cholin, PABA
Maximum Cure Time: 2 Hours

Hanging Skin—as a result of aging or weight loss.

Essential: Molybdenum
Helpful: Vitamins B complex, C, K, bioflavonoids, lipase, rutin, protase, SOD, chromium, germanium, iodine, iron, magnesium, manganese, phosphorus, potassium, vanadium, sodium, selenium, silicon, barley grass, brewers' yeast, gums/mucilages, garlic, green magma, lecithin, octacosanol, spriulina, wheat germ, alfalfa, black cohosh, black walnut, bladder wrack, blue cohosh, catnip, celery seed, chickweed, cornsilk, damiana, dandelion, dong quai, Echinacea, fever-

few, gentian, germander, gingko balboa, Siberian ginseng, grindelia, hawthorn berries, hops, horehound, huckleberries, Irish moss, juniper berries, kelp, licorice root, lobelia, milkweed, nettle, parsley, peppermint, psyllium, pumpkin, red clover, red raspberry, sarsparilla, skullcap, slippery elm, uva ursi, valarian, rose hips
Maximum Cure Time: 2 Years

Hangover

Essential: L-asparagine
Helpful: Vitamin E, bromelin, trypsin, ehymotrypsin, capsicum, Irish moss
Maximum Cure Time: 5 Minutes

Haunta Virus

Essential: Vitamin B-12
Helpful: Vitamins B-2, B-3, B-5, biotin, copper, germanium, iodine, iron, magnesium, manganese, molybdenum, phosphorus, potassium, selenium, silicon, sodium, sulfur, vanadium, zinc, all enzymes, all ammo acids, acidophilus, barley grass, bee pollen/honey, bee propolis, desiccated liver, garlic, green magma, lecithin, octacosanol, spirulina, wheat germ, yarrow, yerbamate, yellow dock, sarsparilla, rose hips, rhubarb root, red raspberry, red clover, pumpkin, psyllium, peppermint, pennyroyal, pau d'arco, parsley, nettle, mullein, alfalfa, chaparral, chickweed, coltsfoot, comfrey root, damiana, dandelion, eyebright, fenugreek, feverfew, flaxseed, gentian, ginger, ginkgo biloba, Siberian ginseng, licorice root, lobelia, milk thistle, milkweed
Maximum Cure Time: 2 Weeks

Headache

Essential: Catalase
Helpful: Calcium, chromium, copper, iron, magnesium, manganese, phosphorus, potassium, selenium, silicon, sodium, sulfur, vanadium, zinc, protase, SOD, spirulina, feverfew, ginger, gingko biloba
Maximum Cure Time: 9 Minutes
This will not work for Sinus, Migraine or tension headaches (Stress).

Heart, Arrhythmias

Essential: Cholin

Helpful: Germanium, Vitamin B-5, biotin, all amino acids, brewers yeast, chlorophyll, evening primrose oil, green magma, slippery elm, uva ursi, white oak bark
Maximum Cure Time: 3 Months

Heart, Congestive Heart Failure and Ischemic Heart Disease

Essential: Coenzyme Q1O
Helpful: Desiccated liver, Irish moss, lobelia, yarrow
Maximum Cure Time: 8 Months

Heart, Fibrillation

Essential: L-Aspartic acid
Helpful: L-Citruline, biotin, spirulina, fennel
Maximum Cure Time: 2 Months

Heart, Ischemic Heart Disease same as Heart, Congestive Heart Failure
Heart, Myocardial Infarction same as Angina Pectoris
Heartburn

Essential: Vitamin B-5
Helpful: Vitamins B-2, B-6, B-12, biotin, cholin, inositol, PABA, all minerals, L-cysteine, L-cystine, GABA, L-glutamine, L-glutathine, L-valine, acidophilus, chlorophyll, garlic, catnip, alfalfa, bladder wrack
Maximum Cure Time: 6 Minutes

Heat Exhaustion

Essential: Potassium
Helpful: Coenzyme Q10, zinc, L~lysine, slippery elm, valarian, yerbamate, Echinacea, fennel, goldenseal, horehound, juniper berries
Maximum Cure Time: 15 Minutes

Hemangioma

Essential: GABA
Helpful: Vanadium, zinc, L-citruline, L-cystine, L-cysteine, L-phenylalaine, DL-phenylalaine, L-leucine, L-methionine, L-ornithine, L-alaine, L-arginine, L-aspartic acid, calendula, capsicum, uva ursi, wtercress, white oak bark, wood betony, yarrow, barley grass, lecithan, octacosanol
Maximum Cure Time: 1 Year

Hemochromatosis

Essential: Manganese
Helpful: Coenzyme Q10, cholin, inositol, PABA, papain, chymotrypsin, lipase, amylase, protase, rutin, catalase, SOD, trypsin, phosphorus, potassium, selenium, silicon, vanadium, zinc, GABA, L-glutathine, L-valine, L-phenylalaine, L-tryptophan, L-tryosine, acidophilus, aloe vera, bee propolis, cellulose, chlorella, chlorophyll, wheat germ, lecithin, octacosanol, green magma, gums/mucilages, white oak bark, yarrow, yucca, celery seed, chickweed, comfrey root, damiana, dandelion, ginger, hops, horehound, huckleberries, juniper berries, licorice root, lobelia, milkweed
Maximum Cure Time: 2 Years

Hemophilia

Essential: Folic acid
Helpful: Vitamins B-3, B-5, B-6, biotin, cholin, PABA, copper, iodine, manganese
Maximum Cure Time: 6 Weeks

Hemorrhoids

Essential: L-Glycine
Helpful: Vitamins A, D, zinc, L-citruline, L-cysteine, L-cystine, L-glutamic acid, L-histidine, L-isoleucine-L-lysine, L-methionine, L-ornithine, L-proline, L-serine, L-taurine, L-tryosine, L-leucine, cellulose, chlorella, catnip, celery seed, corn silk, damiana, hawthorn berries, huckleberries, juniper berries, yarrow
Maximum Cure Time: 1 Day

Hepatitis, Type A

Essential: SOD
Helpful: Vitamins B-l, B-6, D, K, B complex, biotin, folic acid, inositol, bromelin, trypsin, lipase, amylase, protase, catalase, all amino acids, octacosanol, spiraling, blue cohosh, butcher's broom, lobelia
Maximum Cure Time: 8 Weeks

Hepatitis, Type B

Essential: Vitamin A
Helpful: All amino acids, Vitamins B-2, B-3, B-5, B-6, C, D, bioflavonoids, coenzyme Q10, biotin, cholin, inositol, lecithin, wheat germ, yerbamate, dong quai, capsicum
Maximum Cure Time: 7 Weeks

Hepatitis, Type C

Essential: Sulfur
Helpful: All amino acids, all vitamins, zinc, spirulina, horsetail, huckleberries
Maximum Cure Time: 6 Months

Herpes, Type I

Essential: Folic acid
Helpful: Vitamins B-l, B-2, B-3, B-5, B-6, B-12, PABA
Maximum Cure Time: 8 Weeks

Herpes, Type II

Essential: Iodine
Helpful: Boron, calcium, chromium, copper, germanium, iron, magnesium, phosphorus, lipase, amylase, catalase, SOD, all amino acids
Maximum Cure Time: 9 Months Type II herpes is genital.

Hiatal Hernia

Essential: Calcium

Helpful: Chromium, copper, germanium, iodine, iron, magnesium, selenium, silicon, sodium, sulfur, zinc, L-asparagine, L-aspartic acid, L-carnitine, L-cystine, GABA, L-glutamic acid, L-glutamine, L-glutathine, L-valine, L-glycine, L-histidine, L-isoleucine, L-leucine, L-phenylalaine, DL-phenylalaine, L-proline, L-serine, L-taurine, L-threonine, coenzyme Q10
Maximum Cure Time: 8 Months

Hiccups

Essential: L-Methionine
Helpful: Cornsilk
Maximum Cure Time: 2 Minutes

High Blood Pressure

Essential: Potassium
Helpful: Boron, calcium, copper, iodine, iron, magnesium, manganese, molybdenum, phosphorus, L-threonine, L-taurine, L-serine, L-proline, L-ornithine, L-methionine, L-lysine, L-leucine, L-isoleucine, L-histidine, L-glycine, L-alanine, L-arginine, L-asparagine, L-aspartic acid, L-carnitine, L-cystine, L-glutamic acid, L-glutamine, L-glutathine, feverfew, comfrey root, germander, Siberian ginseng, skullcap, suma, valerian
Maximum Cure Time: 8 Days

High Cholesterol

Essential: Coenzyme Q10
Helpful: Manganese, potassium, sulfur, yarrow, yerbamate
Maximum Cure Time: 2 Months

HIV-AIDS

Essential: Magnesium
Helpful: Coenzyme Q10, chromium, wheat germ, cascara sagrada
Maximum Cure Time: 2 Years

Hives

Essential: Sulfur

Helpful: Vitamin B-12, catalase, SOD, vanadium, L-asparagine, L-arginine, L-aspartic acid, bee propolis, cellulose, lecithin, wheat germ, horehound, huckleberries, juniper berries, kelp, uva ursi
Maximum Cure Time: 1 Hour

Hot Flashes

Essential: Copper
Helpful: Vitamins C, K, papain, lipase, protase, zinc
Maximum Cure Time: 4 Months

Huntington's Disease

Essential: L-Taurine
Helpful: Bioflavonoids, L-proline, L-serine, L-tryptophan, octacosanol, horehound, elderberry (fruit)
Maximum Cure Time: 6 Months

Hyperthyroid

Essential: All amino acids
Helpful: Vitamins B-1, B-2, B-3, B-5, B-6, B-12, biotin, cholin, folic acid, inositol, PABA, SOD, vanadium
Maximum Cure Time: 9 Days

Hypoglycemia

Essential: L-Carnitine
Helpful: All minerals, SOD, bioflavonoids, L-cystine
Maximum Cure Time: 6 Weeks

Hypothyroid

Essential: Lipase
Helpful: Vitamins B-1, B-2, B-3, B-5, B-6, B-12, C, D, E, biotin, cholin, folic acid, inositol, PABA, bromelin, papain, tryosine, chymotrypsin, amylase, catalase, protase, all minerals, L-cysteine, L-glycine, L-histidine, L-isoleucine, L-leucine, L-lysine, L-methionine, L-ornithine, DL-phenylalaine, GABA, L-proline,

L-serine, L-taurine, L-threonine, evening primrose oil, yarrow, yucca, nettle, juniper berries
Maximum Cure Time: 3 Months

Impotence

Essential: Folic acid
Helpful: Vitamins A, C, D, E, K, B-l, B-2, B-3, B-5, B-6, B-12, inositol, PABA, L-carnitine, L-cystine, GABA, L-glutamic acid, L-glutamine, L-glutathine, L-glycine, L-histidine, L-isoleucine, L-lysine, L-serine, yerbamate
Maximum Cure Time: 6 Days

Indigestion

Essential: Calcium
Helpful: L-histidine, L-leucine, selenium, iodine, iron, magnesium, phosphorus, potassium, pancreatic NF, bromelin, papain
Maximum Cure Time: 10 Minutes

Infertility

Essential: Boron
Helpful: Silicon, sodium, zinc, chromium, copper, germanium, iodine, iron, magnesium, manganese, molybdenum, phosphorus, potassium, papain, tyrosine, chymotrypsin, L-cysteine, lipase, amylase, rutin, catalase, protase
Maximum Cure Time: 5 Weeks

Inflammation

Essential: L-Cystine
Helpful: All minerals, L-serine, L-taurine, L-threonine, L-tryptophan, L-tyrosine, L-carnitine, L-cysteine, L-glutamic acid, L-glutamine
Maximum Cure Time: 6 Days

Influenza see Flu
Insomnia

Essential: All minerals

Helpful: All enzymes, biotin, cholin, folic acid, inositol, PABA, L-histidine, L-isoleucine, L-leucine, L-lysine, L-aspartic acid, L-carnitine, L-citruline, L-cysteine, L-cystine, L-glutamic acid, L-glutamine, L-glutathine, L-valine, and physical exercise
Maximum Cure Time: 2 Days

Irritable Bowel Syndrome

Essential: PABA
Helpful: Vanadium, phosphorus, L-glutamine, L-glutathine, L-valine, spriulina, wheat germ, licorice root
Maximum Cure Time: 7 Weeks

Jaundice

Essential: L-Ornithine
Helpful: All minerals, all enzymes, L-aspartic acid, L-carnitine, L-citruline, L-cysteine, L-glutamine, L-glutathine, L-valine, L-glycine, L-histidine, L-isoleucine, L-leucine, L-lysine, L-methionine, L-phenylalaine, L-proline, L-serine, L-taurine, L-threonine, L-tryosine
Maximum Cure Time: 6 Hours

Jet Lag

Essential: L-Cysteine
Helpful: L-Citruline, L-cystine
Maximum Cure Time: 1 Hour

Kidney and Bladder Problems

Essential: Vanadium
Helpful: Iron, magnesium, manganese, molybdenum, phosphorus, potassium, selenium, silicon, sodium, sulfur, zinc, papain, trypsin, chymotrypsin, lipase, amylase, rutin, catalase, SOD, protase, Vitamins B-1, B-2, B-5, B-6, B-12, E, K, biotin, cholin, bioflavonoids, coenzyme Q10, folic acid, inositol, PABA, all amino acids, blessed thistle, alfalfa
Maximum Cure Time: 6 Days

Kidney Disease

Essential: SOD
Helpful: Germanium, manganese, potassium, sulfur, L-serine, wheat germ, alfalfa, cascara sagrada, hops, nettle, parsley, rose hips, black cohosh
Maximum Cure Time: 2 Years

Kidney Stones

Essential: Vitamin K
Helpful: Vitamins A, B complex, C, D, bioflavonoids, coenzyme Q10, all B vitamins, chymotrypsin, lipase, amylase, rutin, catalase, SOD, protase, all minerals, L-histidine, L-leucine, L-methionine, DL-phenylalaine, L-proline, L-serine, L-taurine, L-threonine, L-tryptophan, L-tryosine, L-alanine, L-arginine, L-asparagine, L-aspartic acid, L-carnitine, L-citruline, L-cystine, L-glutamic acid, L-glutamine, L-glutathine, L-valine, alfalfa
Maximum Cure Time: 2 Weeks

Lactose Intolerance

Essential: Trypsin
Helpful: Vitamins B complex, E
Maximum Cure Time: 1 Month

Lead Poisoning

Essential: Biotin
Helpful: Vitamins E, B-1, B-2, B-3, B-5, B-1 2, bioflavonoids, coenzyme Q10, eholin, folic acid, inositol, PABA, protase, pancreatin NF, bromelin, papain, trypsin, chymotrypsin, lipase, amylase, rutin, zinc, sodium, silicon, selenium, germanium, iodine, iron, magnesium, manganese, molybdenum, phosphorus, potassium, L-cysteine, L-cystine, L-alanine, GABA, L-glutamic acid, L-glutamine, L-glutathine, L-valine, L-gylcine, L-histidine, L-isoleucine, L-lysine, DL-phenylalaine, L-phenylalaine, L-proline, L-serine, L-taurine, L-threonine, L-tryptophan, L-tryosine, brewers' yeast, bee pollen/honey, parsley, rhubarb root, pennyroyal, horsetail, jumper berries, lobelia
Maximum Cure Time: 9 Days

Legionnaires' Disease

Essential: Coenzyme Q10
Helpful: Vitamin B complex, protase, Siberian ginseng
Maximum Cure Time: 6 Months

Legs, Restless

Essential: Vitamin E
Helpful: Vitamins D, F, bioflavonoids, coenzyme Q10, boron, iron, zinc, L-cysteine, L-cystine, cellulose, capsicum
Maximum Cure Time: 4 Hours
Restless legs always indicate some sort of thyroid problem.

Leg Ulcers

Essential: Vitamin B-5
Helpful: L-Asparagine, L-citruline, L-cysteine, L-glutamic acid, L-glutamine, L-glutathine, L-valine, chlorella, lobelia
Maximum Cure Time: 2 Months

Leukorrhea

Essential: Manganese
Helpful: Vitamins B-2, B-6, B-12, C, E, cholin, folic acid, inositol, PABA, chromium, germanium, phosphorus, all amino acids, capsicum, catnip, sarsaparilla, yarrow, yellow dock
Maximum Cure Time: 2 Months

Leukoderma *see* Vitiligo
Lou Gerhig's Disease (ALS)

Essential: Bioflavonoids
Helpful: Coenzyme Q10, chymotrypsin, protase, amylase, lipase, rutin, catalase, SOD, all minerals, L-glycine, L-isoleucine, L-lysine, L-methionine, L-ornithine, evening primrose oil, Pau d' arco, peppermint, skullcap
Maximum Cure Time: 5 Years

Lupus

Essential: PABA
Helpful: Vitamin B-6, biotin, cholin, folic acid, inositol, all minerals, bromelin, papain, lipase, protase, trypsin, chymotrypsin, rutin, SOD, all amino acids, barley grass, wheat germ, spirulina, green magma, brewers' yeast, peppermint, lobelia, milkweed, ginger, ginkgo biloba, Siberian ginseng, goldenseal, damiana, coenzyme Q10
Maximum Cure Time: 2 Years

Lyme Disease

Essential: Vitamin D
Helpful: Zinc, vanadium, silicon, selenium, calcium, germanium, molybdenum, phosphorus, potassium, papain, trypsin, chymotrypsin, lecithin, wheat germ, suma, yellow dock, yucca, alfalfa, bladderwrack, horsetail, hops, grindelia, garlic
Maximum Cure Time: 2 Months

Mad Cow Disease (CJD)

Essential: Coenzyme Q10
Helpful: Vitamin K, zinc, sulfur, silicon, chromium, copper, germanium, iron, magnesium, manganese, phosphorus, potassium, L-alanine, L-asparagine, L-aspartic acid, L-citruline, L-cystine, GAB A, L-valine, L-proline, L-serine, L-taurine, L-threonine, L-tryptophan, L=phenylalaine, L-glycine, astralagus, chaparral
Maximum Cure Time: 2 Months

Malabsorption Syndrome

Essential: Boron
Helpful: PABA, folic acid, iron, manganese, all amino acids
Maximum Cure Time: 1 Week

Malaria

Essential: Bioflavonoids
Helpful: Octacosanol, acidophilus, chlorella, evening primrose oil, skullcap, slippery elm, thyme, yarrow

Maximum Cure Time: 5 Months

Marburg *see* Ebola

Measles

Essential: Folic acid
Helpful: Cholin, vitamins B-12, B-6, B-2, protase, trypsin, SOD, rutin, L-alanine, L-arginine, L-aspartic acid, L-carnitine, L-cysteine, GABA, L-glutamic acid, L-glutamine, L-glutathine, L-valine, L-glycine, L-histidine, L-isoleucine, DL-phenylalaine, L-proline, L-serine, L-taurine, L-threonine, L-tryptophan, L-tryosine, cellulose, chlorophyll
Maximum Cure Time: 7 Hours
Patient will still be contagious for 2 more days.

Meniere's Syndrome—Ringing of the Ears

Essential: Vitamin B-5
Helpful: Vitamins B complex, B-l, B-6, inositol, cholin, folic acid, calcium, germanium, iron, manganese, potassium, zinc, vanadium, sulfur, pancreatin NF, bromelin, lipase, rutin, chymotrypsin, L-alanine, L-asparagine, L-carnitine, L-citruline, GABA, L-valine, L-phenylalaine, L-serine, L-threonine, copper, brewer's yeast, chlorella, wheat germ, gums/mucilages, chaparral, chickweed, damiana, fennel, feverfew
Maximum Cure Time: 2 Weeks

Meningitis

Essential: Inositol
Helpful: Vitamins A, C, D, E, B-2, B-3, folic acid, PABA, bioflavonoids, trypsin, lipase, amylase, rutin, zinc, catalase, protase, selenium, boron, calcium, copper, germanium, iodine, manganese, magnesium, molybdenum, phosphorus, all amino acids, capsicum, cascara sagrada, catnip
Maximum Cure Time: 2 Months

Menstrual Cramps

Essential: Bioflavonoids
Helpful: Phosphorus, rutin, licorice root, pumpkin, red raspberry

Maximum Cure Time: 20 Minutes

Mercury Toxicity

Essential: Trypsin
Helpful: All amino acids, Vitamins C, D, E, K, B-l, B-2, B-3, B-5, B-6, bioflavonoids, cholin, folic acid, inositol, PABA, all minerals except selenium, sodium, and vanadium, octacosanol
Maximum Cure Time: 2 Months

Migraine

Essential: Zinc
Helpful: Bromelin, papain, trypsin, amylase, L-carnitine, L-leucine, L-threonine
Maximum Cure Time: 2 Hours

Mononucleosis

Essential: Vanadium
Helpful: Vitamin B-l2, folic acid, phosphorus, green magma, grindelia, lobelia
Maximum Cure Time: 5 Weeks

Morgallons Disease

Essential: Vitamin A
Helpful: Vitamin E, bioflavonoids, iodine, magnesium, molybdenum, sodium, sulfur, vanadium, L-carnitine, L-cysteine, L-glutamic acid, L-histidine, L-lysine, L-methionine, DL-phenylalaine, L-tryosine, lecithin, chamomile, comfrey root, corn silk, kelp, licorice root, rhubarb root, rose hips, sarsaparilla, thyme, uva ursi, watercress, yellow dock, yucca
Maximum Cure Time: 3 Weeks

Motion Sickness

Essential: Coenzyme Q10
Helpful: Ginger
Maximum Cure Time: 30 Minutes

Multiple Sclerosis and Muscular Dystrophy

Essential: Inositol
Helpful: Vitamins B-5, B-6, B-12, K, cholin, L-histidine, L-isoleucine, DL-phenylalaine, L-serine, L-taurine, L-threonine, L-valine
Maximum Cure Time: 8 Months

Mumps

Essential: Vitamin F
Helpful: Vitamins B complex, C, E, L-ornithine, L-tryosine, gums/mucilages, valerian, milkweed, evening primrose oil
Maximum Cure Time: 8 Days

Muscle Cramps

Essential: GABA
Helpful: Folic acid, calcium, chromium, copper, iron, manganese, selenium, sulfur, sodium, vanadium, zinc, L-carnitine, L-citruline, L-glutamic acid, L-isoleucine, L-proline, L-serine, L-threonine, astralagus, calendula, chaparral, chickweed, eyebright, feverfew, huckleberries, juniper berries, kelp, nettle, parsley, psyllium, red clover, red raspberry, rhubarb root, rose hips, sarsaparilla, suma, thyme, uva ursi, valerian, watercress, white oak bark, wood betony, yarrow, yerbamate
Maximum Cure Time: 20 Minutes

Muscular Dystrophy *see* Multiple Sclerosis
Muscles and Joints

Essential: All enzymes
Helpful: Vitamins B complex, C, E, F, coenzyme Q10, copper, magnesium, potassium, selenium, L-glycine, L-isoleucine, L-leucine, L-lysine, GABA, L-threonine, cellulose, spirulina, gums/mucilages, lecithin, rhubarb root, sarsaparilla, slippery elm, uva ursi, valerian, buchu, capsicum, catnip, chamomile, comfrey root, flaxseed, horsetail, juniper berries, licorice root, lobelia
Maximum Cure Time: 5 Hours

Myalgia

Essential: SOD
Helpful: Rutin, L-leucine, DL-phenylalaine, chlorella, chorophyll, desiccated liver, gums/mucilages, garlic, lecithin, octacosanol, butcher's broom, capsicum, gotu kola, peppermint, uva ursi, skullcap
Maximum Cure Time: 4 Years

Nagging Cough

Essential: Vitamin A
Helpful: Vitamins C, B-5, B-6, coenzyme Q10, cholin, inositol, bromelin, papain, trypsin, rutin, catalase, SOD, L-aspartic acid, L-citruline, L-isoleucine, L-methionine, L-ornithine, L-tryosine, lecithin, octacosanol, wheat germ, garlic, chamomile, chaparral, coltsfoot, comfrey root, cornsilk, damiana, dandelion, dong quay, fennel, fenugreek, germander, ginger, gingko biloba, Siberian ginseng, goldenseal, gotu kola, hawthorn berries, hops, horehound, horsetail, huckleberries, Irish moss, juniper berries, kelp, lobelia, milkweed, nettle, parsley, peppermint, psyllium, pumpkin, red raspberry, rosehips, sarsaparilla, eyebright
Maximum Cure Time: 1 Hour

Nail Biting

Essential: L-Serine
Helpful: L-Taurine
Maximum Cure Time: 3 days

Nail Picking

Essential: L-Alanine
Helpful: Coenzyme Q10, manganese, phosphorus, copper, sodium, sulfur, vanadium, L-carnitine, L-citruline
Maximum Cure Time: 3 days

Nail Problems

Essential: Calcium
Helpful: Vitamin B complex, PABA
Maximum Cure Time: 2 Months

Nausea

Essential: L-Methionine
Helpful: L-Histidine, ginger
Maximum Cure Time: 10 Minutes

Nose Bleeds

Essential: Boron
Helpful: Siberian ginseng, white oak bark
Maximum Cure Time: 5 Minutes

Obesity

Essential: Iodine
Helpful: Vitamin E, silicon, all amino acids, milk thistle
Weight loss will be slow and gradual—months to years to achieve normal weight depending up on obesity.

Osteoporosis

Essential: Vitamin D
Helpful: Nettles
Maximum Cure Time: 8 Months

Pain from Injury

Essential: Chymotrypsin
Helpful: Vitamins A, B-6, B-12, cholin, folic acid inositol, PABA, boron, calcium, chromium, germanium, iodine, iron, green magma, celery seed, chickweed, coltsfoot, damiana, dandelion, hips, lobelia, peppermint, yerbamate, spirulina
Maximum Cure Time: 2 Hours

Pancreatitis

Essential: Zinc
Helpful: Trypsin, chromium, copper, evening primrose oil, green magma, fenugreek

Maximum Cure Time: 14 Days

Parkinson's Disease

Essential: Vitamin A
Helpful: Vitamins B-l, B-2, B-3, B-6, B-12, cholin, folic acid, all minerals, all amino acids, green magma, capsicum, coltsfoot, skullcap, fenugreek, feverfew, damiana, alfalfa, barberry, black cohosh, black walnut, bladderwrack, blessed thistle, blue cohosh, blue vervain, buchu, burdock root butcher's broom
Maximum Cure Time: 2 Years

Pellagra

Essential: Coenzyme Q1O
Helpful: Vitamins B-5, B-12, biotin, cholin, garlic, wheat germ
Maximum Cure Time: 2 Years

Periodontal Disease

Essential: Vitamin K
Helpful: Alfalfa
Maximum Cure Time: 5 Months

Phlebitis

Essential: Phosphorus
Helpful: Vitamins E, F, K, bioflavonoids, coenzyme Q10, folic acid, copper, L-phenylalaine, DL-phenylalaine, L-proline, L-serine, L-taurine, L-threonine, L-tryptophan, L-tryosine, cellulose, desiccated liver, evening primrose oil, alfalfa
Maximum Cure Time: 10 Weeks

Pneumonia

Essential: Vitamin K
Helpful: Vitamins D, E, bioflavonoids, papain, chymotrypsin
Maximum Cure Time: 10 Days

Poison Ivy

Essential: Vitamin B-12
Helpful: Vitamins C, E, F, B-6, cholin, inositol, bromelin, papain, trypsin, chymotrypsin, catalase, milk thistle, juniper berries
Maximum Cure Time: 5 Days

Poison Oak

Essential: L-Glutamic acid
Helpful: Bromelin, amylase, catalase, L-citruline, L-glutathine, L-valine
Maximum Cure Time: 1 Day

Polio

Essential: Zinc***
Helpful: Vitamins C, E, all amino acids, octacosonal, thyme, peppermint, horehound, lobelia
Maximum Cure Time: 4 Years
***Physicians should give zinc in the form of injections ONLY.

Premature Births

Some pregnant women **May** benefit from **ONE** of the following: Germanium, garlic, octacosanol, spirulina, wheat germ, gotu kola, hops, juniper berries, fennel, germander. Either muscle test or dowse to determine if any is needed. Take for a **MAXIMUM** of 2 weeks **ONLY** during the first trimester.

Premenstrual Syndrome

Essential: All amino acids
Helpful: Zinc, acidophilus, bee pollen/honey, bee propolis, brewers' yeast, cellulose, chlorella, chlorophyll, evening primrose oil, lecithin, octacosanol, spirulina, wheat germ, nettle, parsley, pau d'arco, pennyroyal, peppermint, red clover, red raspberry, rhubarb root, rose hips, slippery elm, suma, thyme, uva ursi, valerian, watercress, white oak bark, yarrow, black cohosh, blessed thistle, blue cohosh, buchu, burdock root, butcher's broom, cascara sagrada, chamomile, comfrey root, fennel, fenugreek, feverfew, flaxseed, gentian, ginger, ginkgo biloba, Siberian ginseng, goldenseal, huckleberries, Irish moss, juniper berries

Maximum Cured Time: 5 Hours

Psoriasis

Essential: All enzymes
Helpful: Vitamins A, B complex, C, D, E, F, K, bioflavonoids, zinc, L-isoleucine, L-methionine, DL-phenylalaine, L-proline, L-serine, L-taurine, L-threonine, L-tryptophan, L-tryosine, comfrey root, suma, uva ursi, yellow dock, yucca
Maximum Cure Time: 2 Months

Rabidity—Bitten by Rabid Animals

Essential: Sodium
Adults need to take 1/2 teaspoon of salt in water 8 times in 24 hours. For children the amount of salt should be reduced to 1/4 teaspoon per dose.

Radiation Poisoning

Essential: Chymotrypsin
Helpful: Vitamins A, D, E, bioflavonoids, lipase, trypsin, sulfur, zinc, barley grass, garlic, lecithin, chlorophyll, celery seed, chaparral, coltsfoot, damiana, goldenseal, hops, horehound, huckleberries, milk thistle, yellow dock, yucca
May also need to have supplemental thyroid up to 60mg/day for adults and 20mg/day for children 12 and under. Check blood levels.
Maximum Cure Time: 3 Months

Raynaud's Disease

Essential: Bioflavonoids
Helpful: Vitamins E, K, wheat germ, bladderwrack, cornsilk, comfrey root, buchu, lobelia
Maximum Cure Time: 5 Years

Reye's Syndrome

Essential: Coenzyme Q10
Helpful: Vitamin B-2, pancreatin, bromelin, papain, amylase, rutin, zinc, sulfur, sodium, vanadium, calcium, iodine, iron, magnesium, manganese, molybdenum, phosphorus, potassium, L-alanine, L-arginine, L-cysteine, L-carnitine, L-cit-

ruline, L-glutathine, L-valine, L-glycine, L-isoleucine, L-methionine, L-ornithine, DL-phenylalaine, L-proline, L-serine, wheat germ, spirulina, barley grass
Maximum Cure Time: 5 Months

Rheumatic Fever

Essential: Vitamin B complex
Helpful: Vitamin C, comsilk
Maximum Cure Time: 6 Days

Rickets

Essential: Vitamin C
Helpful: Vitamin D, bioflavonoids, PABA, iron, magnesium, selenium, silicon,
L-glutamic acid, damiana, milk thistle
Maximum Cure Time: 2 Years

Rocky Mountain Fever

Essential: Vitamin D
Helpful: Vitamin K, coenzyme Q10, selenium, sulfur, zinc, vanadium, calcium,
chromium, copper, L-aspartic acid, L-carnitine, L-citruline, L-cysteine, L-cystine,
GABA, L-glutamic acid, L-glutamine, L-glutathine, L-valine, L-histidine, L-isoleucine, L-leucine, L-lysine, L-methionine, L-ornithine, L-phenylalaine, DL-phenylalaine, L-serine, L-taurine, L-tryosine, gums/mucilages, garlic, green magma,
sarsaparilla
Maximum Cure Time: 2 Days
This virus is carried by mosquitoes. Within one hour of bite, patient will have a
fever over 100 degrees F.
Persons with adequate Vitamin D in their systems will be unaffected.

RSV

Essential: Protase
Helpful: Green magma
Maximum Cure Time: 4 Minutes
This is a deadly disease that sometimes occurs in infants but looks like a simple
cold. If you think your infant has a cold, give the child pineapple juice or fruit,

depending upon age. If the child has RSV, it will clear up within the 4 minutes. If it does not clear up, treat for a cold. A child can die of RSV within 5 minutes.

Scabies

Essential: Vitamin B complex
Helpful: Vitamins B-l, B-2, B-3, B-6, folic acid, PABA, papain, rutin, protase, catalase, SOD, boron, calcium, manganese, molybdenum, phosphorus, potassium, sodium, silicon, sulfur, vanadium, L-aspartic acid, L-citruline, L-cysteine, L-cystine, L-glutamic acid, L-glutamine, L-glutathine, L-histidine, L-leucine, L-ornithine, L-phenylalaine, DL-phenylalaine, L-proline, L-serine, L-taurine, L-tryptophan, L-tryosine, bee propolis, green magma, octacosanol, spirulina, wheat germ, black cohosh, blessed thistle, blue cohosh, blue vervain, buchu, catnip, chamomile, chaparral, chickweed, coltsfoot, comfrey root, damiana, dandelion, horehound, horsetail, Irish moss, kelp, licorice root, lobelia, milk thistle, pennyroyal, skullcap, slippery elm, suma, thyme, uva ursi, valerian, watercress, wood betony
Maximum Cure Time: 6 Weeks

Scarring

Essential: Inositol
Helpful: Coenzyme Q10, Vitamin B-6, trypsin, green magma, lecithin, octacosanol, catnip
Maximum Cure Time: 1 Week

Seborrhea

Essential: Selenium
Helpful: Vitamins C, D, PABA, copper, zinc, aloe vera, gums/mucilages, green magma, gotu kola, nettle, red clover, yucca valerian, thyme
              Chickweed may be used EXTERNALLY ONLY
Maximum Cure Time: 3 Weeks

Shingles

Essential: L-Lysine
Helpful: Coenzyme Q10
Maximum Cure Time: 19 Days

Author's Note: Many years ago I received directions to cure shingles from my sister who got it from a friend. I was over them by the time I received the directions but passed them on to an elderly friend who found it successful: On day 1, take one pill of L-lysine, on day 2, take 2 and so on until you feel relief. Then stay at that number of pills each day until the shingles are clearly gone. At that point, reverse the order, taking one less pill each day until you are taking none. Avoid chocolate and nuts until cured.

Sickle-cell Anemia

Essential: Vitamin B-12
Helpful: Vitamins B-2, C, K, coenzyme Q10, all amino acids, green magma, suma, buchu, hawthorn berries
Maximum Cure Time: 3 Years
African people require a higher level of B-12 than those of other races.

Sinusitis

Essential: PABA
Helpful: Vitamins B-l, B-2, B-3, B-12, cholin, L-ornithine, octacosanol, spirulina, mullein, pennyroyal, valerian, yucca, huckleberries, Irish moss, astragalus, catnip
Maximum Cure Time: 2 Days

Sleep Apnea

Essential: Iodine
Helpful: Vitamins A, C, D, E, bioflavoniods, catalase, trypsin, pancreatine NF, selenium, iron, manganese, phosphorus, molybdenum, flaxseed, ginger, kelp
Maximum Cure Time: 4 Years
Note: This symptom indicates Blocked Thyroid *See* What To Do If You Have A Blocked Thyroid.

Smallpox

Essential: PABA
Helpful: Vitamins C, E, F, B-l, B-2, cholin, L-methionine, L-ornithine, L-phenylalaine, DL-phenylalaine, L-taurine, L-serine, L-tryptophan, chlorophyll, garlic, sarsaparilla, slippery elm, suma, uva ursi, valerian, watercress, wood betony,

black cohosh, blessed thistle, buchu, cascara sagrada, celery seed, chamomile, chaparral, ehickweed, coltsfoot, cornsilk, dandelion
Maximum Cure Time: 6 Months
If none of the above is available, eat at least 1 cup cooked brown rice per day or 3/4 cup cooked barley per day.

Snake Bite, Non-Poisonous

Essential: Catalase
Helpful: Lipase, yarrow, hops, Irish moss, fennel, feverfew, goldenseal, ginger
Zinc may be use EXTERNALLY ONLY
Maximum Cure Time: 2 Days

Snake Bite, Poisonous

Essential: Vitamin A—Patient should take 10,000 IU as soon as possible!
Helpful: Vitamins C, F, coenzyme Q10, PABA, all enzymes, L-phenylalaine, DL-phenylalaine, L-proline, L-serine, L-taurine, L-threonine, L-tryptophan, L-tryosine, brewers' yeast, evening primrose oil, nettle, grindelia, milkweed
Maximum Cure Time: 2 Hours

Sore Throat

Essential: Vitamin C
Helpful: L-Leucine, rose hips, blue cohosh, burdock root, butcher's broom, calendula, capsicum, cascara sagrada, catnip, chamomile, chaparral, coltsfoot, comfrey root, cornsilk, dandelion, dong quai, echinacea, fennel, fenugreek, feverfew, gentian, goldenseal, gotu kola, hops, horehound
Maximum Cure Time: 1 Hour

Spinal Cord Injury—Paralysis

Essential: Papain
Helpful: Vitamin B complex, all minerals, L-leucine, L-lysine, L-methionine, L-phenylalaine, DL-phenylalaine, L-proline, L-serine, L-taurine, L-threonine, L-tryptophan, L-tryosine, bee pollen/honey, bee propolis, cellulose, desiccated liver, evening primrose oil, green magma, lecithin, spirulina, wheat germ, mullein, nettle, parsley, pau d'arco, pumpkin, milk thistle, astralagus, black walnut, bladderwrack, chaparral, coltsfoot

Maximum Cure Time: 7 Years

Sprains, Strains, and Injuries *see* Muscles and Joints
Stained Teeth

Essential: Catalase
Helpful: Trypsin, black walnut, blue cohosh, horsetail
Maximum Cure Time: 2 Months

Staph

Essential: Coenzyme Q10
Helpful: L-PhenyMaine, DL-Phenylalaine
Maximum Cure Time: 3 Days

Streptococcal (Strep) Infections

Essential: Calendula leaves
Maximum Cure Time: 2 Days

Stress

Essential: Magnesium
Helpful: Bioflavonoids, folic acid, inositol, coenzyme Q10, potassium, zinc, L-glycine, L-methionine, L-ornithine, L-phenylalaine, DL-phenylalaine, L-tryosine, lecithin, cascara sagrada, catnip, celery seed, chamomile
Maximum Cure Time: 1 Day

Stroke

Essential: L-Valine
Helpful: Bee propolis, cellulose, skullcap, yellow dock
Maximum Cure Time: 6 Months

Sunburn

Essential: Coenzyme Q10

Helpful: Vitamins C, D, E, F, K, bioflavonoids, bromelin, chymotrypsin, lipase, amylase, catalase, calcium, germanium, iron, potassium, acidophilus, horsetail, white oak bark, yarrow, yucca, psyllium

Aloe vera and wood betony can be used EXTERNALLY ONLY.

Maximum Cure Time: 1 Hour

Tetanus

Essential: L-Arginine
Helpful: All minerals, green magma, spirulina, wheat germ, barley grass, brewers' yeast, desiccated liver, sarsaparilla, slippery elm, uva ursa, watercress, white oak bark, wood betony, catnip, chamomile, huckleberries, Irish moss, juniper berries, kelp, milk thistle, milk weed
Maximum Cure Time: 2 Hours

TMJ—Temperomandibular Joint Syndrome

Essential: Cholin
Helpful: Amylase, catalase, protase, vanadium, L-cystine, L-glutamic acid, L-proiine, L-threonine, gums/mucilages, aloe vera, bee pollen/honey, bee propolis, chlorophyll, black walnut blue vervain, vitamin B-5
Maximum Cure Time: 2 Weeks

Tonsillitis

Essential: Iodine
Helpful: Vitamins B-5, B-12, biotin, papain, copper, phosphorus, potassium, vanadium, all amino acids, aloe vera, barley grass, bee pollen/honey, bee propolis, brewers' yeast, garlic, green magma, octacosanol, spirulina, wheat germ, rose hips, rhubarb root, red clover, uva ursi, watercress, valerian, white oak bark, yarrow, yellow dock, yerbamate, yucca, capsicum, cascara sagrada, celery seed, chamomile, chickweed, comfrey root, echinacea, fennel, fenugreek, feverfew, ginkgo biloba, Siberian ginseng, goldenseal
Maximum Cure Time: 2 Weeks

Triglycerides, High

Essential: Vitamin A
Helpful: Cellulose, evening primrose oil, Siberian ginseng, calendula, damiana

Maximum Cure Time: 8 Weeks

Tuberculosis

Essential: Silicon
Helpful: Vitamins A, C, D, K, slippery elm, watercress, white oak bark, fennel, gentian, Siberian ginseng, horsetail
Maximum Cure Time: 6 Weeks

Tumors

Essential: Pancreatin NF
Helpful: Folic acid, SOD, zinc, catnip, yellow dock
Maximum Cure Time: 2 Months

Typhoid

Essential: Vitamin A
Helpful: Vitamins B complex, C, chlorella
Maximum Cure Time: 2 Months

Ulcers

Essential: Protase
Helpful: Pancreatin NF, L-asparagine, L-citruline, L-cystine, L-glutamine, L-glutathine, L-valine, L-glycine, L-histidine, GABA, aloe vera, evening primrose oil, octacosanol, lecithin, gums/mucilages, catnip, chamomile, Irish moss
Maximum Cure Time: 7 Weeks

Underweight

Essential: Sodium
Helpful: Selenium, all amino acids
Maximum Cure Time: 5 Weeks

Varicose Veins

Essential: Vitamin F

Helpful: Vitamins B complex, C, D, E, vanadium, zinc, chromium, iodine, iron, magnesium, manganese, molybdenum, phosphorus, potassium, cascara sagrada, comfrey root, evening primrose oil, cornsilk, white oak bark, yarrow
Maximum Cure Time: 5 Weeks

Vertigo

Essential: Vitamin B-6
Helpful: Potassium, silicon, sodium, vanadium, zinc
Maximum Cure Time: 4 Hours

Vitiligo/Leukoderma

Essential: Rutin
Helpful: Manganese, germanium
Maximum Cure Time: 5 Years

Warts, Common

Essential: All amino acids
Maximum Cure Time: 8 Days

Warts, Venereal or Genital

Essential: Gentian
Helpful: Vitamin F, fenugreek
Maximum Cure Time: 4 Days—No longer contagious after warts have healed

West Nile Virus

Essential: Bromelin
Helpful: Vitamins A, B complex, B-l, B-2, B-6, B-l 2, D, E, F, coenzyme Q10, biotin, inositol, PABA, rutin
Maximum Cure Time: 6 Weeks

Whooping Cough

Essential: Potassium

Helpful: Vitamins F, C, B-3, B-6, bioflavonoids, inositol, coenzyme Q10, boron, magnesium, manganese, molybdenum, potassium, silicon, vanadium, zinc, L-cysteine, L-citruline, L-arginine, L-carnitine, celery see, alfalfa, evening primrose oil, chlorophyll
Maximum Cure Time: 2 Weeks

Wilson's Disease

Essential: PABA
Helpful: Vitamin B-3, inositol, selenium, sodium, zinc, calcium, chromium, iron, magnesium, manganese, molybdenum, phosphorus, potassium, protase, catalase, damiana, lobelia, horehound, hops
Maximum Cure Time: 8 Weeks

Worms

Essential: Black walnut
Helpful: Horehound, horsetail, uva ursi, watercress, wood betony, yerbamate
Maximum Cure Time: 12 Days

Yeast Infection

Essential: Alfalfa
Helpful: Acidophilus, chlorella, suma, milkweed, cascara sagrada, catnip
Maximum Cure Time: 3 Days

How to Dowse for Cures to Illness

1. Begin by asking "May I, can I, should I dowse for (person in need)?"

2. Request assistance or guidance from the Universal Force.

3. "Does this person have a blocked thyroid?" If no, go to 4.
If yes, patient should refer to What To Do If You Have a Blocked Thyroid.

4. Dowse through the list of nutrients, supplements, and herbs, indicating what the patient needs. (This is easiest if you ask things like "Does the patient need anything listed on this page—in this column," etc. Then go down only the lists indicated).
Vitamins and minerals—dowse how many milligrams (Mg) or micrograms (Mcg)
Vitamins A and E come in International Units (IU)
For all other items, dowse the number of pills the patient should take and the number of times per day. (You will need a chart with numbers for this. If you do not have one, make one.)

5. Finally ask if the patient should take all of the listed items the same length of time and clarify how long for each.

Nutrients, Supplements, Herbs

Vitamins

A

B COMPLEX

C

D

E

F

K

Bioflavonoids

Co Enzyme Q10

B-l Thiamine

B-2 Riboflavin

B-3 Niacin

B-5 Pantothenic Acid

B-6 Pyridoxine

B-12 Cyanocobalamin

Biotin

Cholin

Folic Acid

Inositol

Para-Aminobenzoic Acid
(PABA)

Minerals

Boron

Calcium

Chromium

Copper

Germanium

Iodine

Iron

Magnesium

Manganese

Molybdenum

Phosporus

Potassium

Selenium

Silicon

Sulfur

Vanadium

Zinc

Enzymes

Pancreatine

Bromelin

Papain

Trypsin

Chymotrypsin

Lipase

Amylase

Rutin

Catalase

Superoxide Dismutase
(SOD)

Protase

Amino Acids

L-Alanine

L-Arginine

L-Asparagine

L-Aspartic Acid

L-Carnitine

L-Citruline

L-Cysteine

L-Cystine

Gamma-Aminobutyric Acid (GABA)	Brewers' Yeast	Butcher's Broom
L-Glutamic Acid	Cellulose	Calendula
L-Glutathine	Chlorella	Capsicum
L-Glycine	Chlorophyll	Cascara Sagrada
L-Histidine	Disiccated Liver	Catnip
L-Isoleucine	Evening Primrose Oil	Celery Seed
L-Leucine	Gums/Mucilages	Chamomile
L-Lysine	Garlic	Chaparral
L-Methionine	Green Magma	Chickweed
L-Ornithine	Lecithan	Coltsfoot
L-Phenylalaine	Octacosanol	Comfrey Root
DL-Phenylalaine	Spirulina	Cornsilk
L-Proline	Wheat Germ	Damiana
L-Seirine	**Herbs**	Dandelion
L-Taurine	Alfalfa	Don Quai
L-Threonine	Astragalus	Echinacea
L-Tryptophan	Barberry	Eyebright
L-Tryosine	Black Cohosh	Fennel
L-Valine	Black Walnut	Fenugreek
Supplements	Bladderwrack	Feverfew
Acidophilus/Bifidus	Blessed Thistle	Flaxseed
Aloe Vera	Blue Cohosh	Gentian
Barley Grass	Blue Vervain	Germander
Bee Pollen/Honey	Buchu	Ginger
Bee Propolis	Burdock Root	Ginkgo Biloba

Ginseng (Siberian)

Goldenseal

Gotu Kola

Grindelia

Hawthorn Berries

Hops

Horehound

Horsetail

Huckleberries

Irish Moss

Juniper Berries

Kelp

Licorice Root

Lobelia

Milk Thistle

Milkweed

Mullen

Nettle

Parsley

Pau d' Arco

Pennyroyal

Peppermint

Psyllium

Pumpkin

Red Clover

Red Raspberry

Rhubarb Root

Rose Hips

Sarsaparilla

Skullcap

Slippery Elm

Suma

Thyme

Uva Ursi

Valarian

Watercress

White Oak Bark

Wood Betony

Yarrow

Yellow Dock

Yerbamate

Yucca

Other

Food Sources for Amino Acids

L-Alanine

Cream/butter

Cream cheese

Edam cheese

L-Arginine

Yogurt

Cheddar cheese

Gouda cheese

Provolone cheese

American cheese

L-Asparagine

Garlic

Onions

Celery

Spinach

Arugula

Radicchio

Raw milk

Cottage cheese

Carrots

Hot peppers

Dandelion greens

L-Aspartic Acid

Hot peppers

Pecans

Brazil nuts

Cashews

Blueberries

Boysenberries

Cantaloupe

Cherries

Cranberries

Elderberries

Honeydew

Kiwifruit

Lemons

Pineapple

Raspberries

Rhubarb

Strawberries

L-Carnitine

Kefir

Yogurt

Swiss cheese

Radish

Tomatoes

Eggplant

Radicchio

Sprouts

Tomatillo

Blueberries

Elderberries

Cranberries

Dates

Lemons

Currents

Nectarines

Peaches

Persimmon

Raspberries

Rhubarb

Strawberries

Almonds

English walnuts

Filberts

Brazil nuts

Pistachios

L-Citruline

Cantaloupe

Grapefruit

Gooseberries

Kiwifruit

Lemons

Oranges

Pawpaw

Pineapple

Persimmon

Raspberries

English walnuts

Filberts

Brazil nuts

Cream cheese

Mozzarella cheese

Roquefort cheese

L-Cysteine

Cherries

Elderberries

Gooseberries

Lemons

Mangoes

Pawpaw

Raspberries

Strawberries

Watermelon

Black walnuts

Pine nuts

Millet

Triticale

Barley

Brown rice

Swiss cheese

Gouda cheese

Muenster cheese

Parmesan cheese

Cucumbers

Okra

Peas

Pumpkin

Rutabaga

Mustard greens

Radish

Corn

Popcorn

Lettuce

Arugula

Dandelion greens

Brussels sprouts

Chinese cabbage

Summer squash

L-Cystine

Yogurt

Cream cheese

Apricots

Currents

Peaches

Plums

Cashews

Gamma-Aminobutyric

Acid (GABA)

Cabbage

Okra	Yogurt	Mustard greens
Onions	Kamut	Hot peppers
Spinach	Rye	Broccoli
Radish	Blueberries	Tomatoes
Corn	Cherries	Corn
Popcorn	Cranberries	Chinese cabbage
Dandelion greens	Gooseberries	Eggplant
Brussels sprouts	Figs	String beans
Chinese cabbage	Oranges	
Eggplant		L-Glutathine
Horseradish	L-Glutamine	Carrots
Dry beans	Millet	Celery
Radicchio	Brown rice	Pumpkin
Sprouts	Yogurt	Sweet peppers
Tomatillo	Swiss cheese	Hot peppers
	Blue cheese	Broccoli
L-Glutamic Acid	Brick cheese	Dandelion greens
Cabbage	Colby cheese	Horseradish
Carrots	Gouda cheese	String beans
Spinach	Mozzarella cheese	Soybeans
Sweet potato	Muenster cheese	Quinoa
Cauliflower	American cheese	Millet
Radish	Roquefort cheese	Barley
Horseradish	Spinach	Wild rice
Sprouts	Turnips	Plums

Cantaloupe

Elderberries

Grapefruit

Pawpaw

Nectarines

Pineapple

Raspberries

Rhubarb

Pecans

Cashews

Pistachios

L-Valine

Oats

Wild rice

Brown rice

White rice

Processed milk

Cream/butter

Yogurt

Kefir

Cottage cheese

Provolone cheese

Mozzarella cheese

Cheddar cheese

Cabbage

Cucumber

Garlic

Celery

Okra

Onions

Peas

Pumpkin

Sweet potato

Sweet peppers

Broccoli

Cauliflower

Lettuce

Dandelion greens

Endive Chinese cabbage

String beans

Soybeans

Dry beans

Radicchio

Sprouts

Tomatillo

L-Glycine

Endive

Sprouts

White rice

Apricots

Cherries

Cranberries

Gooseberries

Honeydew

Dates

Kiwifruit

Pawpaw

Pineapple

Persimmon

Strawberries

Watermelon

Black walnuts

Filberts

Cashews

Coconut

L-Isoleucine

Cashews

Coconut

Mozzarella cheese

Muenster cheese

Roquefort cheese

L-Histidine	L-Lysine	Cottage cheese
Lettuce	Artichoke	Yogurt
Sprouts	Onions	Cream cheese
Summer squash	Spinach	Brick cheese
Tomatillo	Corn	Edam cheese
Cottage cheese	Endive	Gouda cheese
Yogurt	String beans	Provolone cheese
Cream cheese	Dry beans	Mozzarella cheese
Colby cheese	Buckwheat	Muenster cheese
Muenster cheese	Wild rice	Parmesan cheese
Roquefort cheese		
Buckwheat	L-Methionine	L-Phenylalaine
White rice	Triticale	Bananas
Peaches	Brown rice	Boysenberries
Pineapple	White rice	Cantaloupe
Raspberries	Oats	Grapes
	Millet	Gooseberries
L-Leucine	Rye	Honeydew
Raw milk		Plums
Cottage cheese	L-Ornithine	Rhubarb
Yogurt	Wheat	Collards
Cream/butter	Kamut	Cucumber
Cream cheese	Quinoa	Celery
Muenster	Oats	Eggplant
	Millet	Peas

Potatoes	Pumpkin	Persimmon
Parsnips	Kefir	Raspberries
Sweet potatoes	Roquefort cheese	Almonds
Sweet peppers		English walnuts
Horseradish	L-Serine	Filberts
Sprouts	Cucumber	Pine nuts
Radicchio	Onions	Brazil nuts
Summer squash	Potatoes	Pistachios
	Pumpkin	
DL-Phenylalaine	Sweet potatoes	L-Taurine
Garlic	Hot peppers	Bananas
Peas	Corn	Cantaloupe
Potatoes	Arugula	Grapefruit
Pumpkins	Endive	Honeydew
Sweet potatoes	Eggplant	Kiwifruit
Sweet peppers	Dry beans	Blueberries
Brown rice	Sprouts	Strawberries
	Summer squash	
L-Proline	Bananas	L-Threonine
Cabbage	Elderberry	Raw milk
Collards	Grapes	Processed milk
Cucumber	Grapefruit	Kefir
Celery	Goose berries	Cream cheese
Okra	Lemons	Brick cheese
Potatoes	Mangoes	Colby cheese

Edam cheese

Provolone cheese

Muenster cheese

Parmesan cheese

L-Tryptophan

Raw milk

Cream/butter

Kefir

Cottage cheese

Brick cheese

Gouda cheese

Provolone cheese

Parmesan cheese

L-Tyrosine

Parsley

Food Sources for Enzymes

Pancreatine NF

Watermelon

Almonds

Filberts

Black walnuts

Pine nuts

Persimmon

Bromeline

Buckwheat

Grapefruit

Lemons

Oranges

Pineapple

Pawpaw

Papain

Cherries

Grapefruit

Pawpaw

Pineapple

Persimmon

Lipase

Bananas

Arugula

Brussels sprouts

Sprouts

Cheddar cheese

Mozzarella

Triticale

Barley

Amylase

Cranberries

Celery

Turnips

Sweet peppers

Arugula

Eggplant

Carrots

Catalase

Okra

Spinach

Hot peppers

Popcorn

Lettuce

Arugula

Soybeans

Blueberries

Boysenberries

Cherries

Grapes

Gooseberries

Nectarines

Raspberries

Protase

Cherries

Elderberries

Figs

Papaya

Pawpaw	Filberts	Sprouts
Pineapple	Cashews	
Plums	Pine nuts	<u>Trypsin</u>
Rhubarb	Coconut	Onions
Buckwheat	Cream/butter	Parsnips
Okra	Brick cheese	Spinach
Pumpkin	Edam cheese	Mustard greens
Spinach	Provolone Parmesan	Sweet peppers
Turnips	American	Hot peppers
Rutabaga	Roquefort	Radish
Radish		Dandelion greens
Corn	<u>Chymotrypsin</u>	Endive
Lettuce	Boysenberries	String beans
Arugula	Persimmon	Persimmon
Endive	Garlic	Raspberries
	Peas	English walnuts
<u>Rutin</u>	Pumpkin/squash	Black walnuts
Apples	Sweet peppers	Brazil nuts
Cranberries	Hot peppers	Coconut
Peaches	Radish	Sprouts
Pineapple	Lettuce	Oats
Rhubarb	Dandelion greens	Critical
Raspberries	Endive	Rye
Watermelon	Brussels sprouts	Lemons
Almonds	Chinese cabbage	Mangoes

Currents

Papaya

Peaches

Pineapple

<u>Superoxide Dismutase</u>

<u>(SOD)</u>

Asparagus

Collards

Peas

Pumpkin/squash

String beans

Lettuce

Rutabaga

Sweet peppers

Cauliflower

Arugula

Brussels sprouts

Eggplant

Soybeans

Radicchio

Black walnuts

Pine nuts

Almonds

Coconut

Blue cheese

Cheddar cheese

American cheese

Rhubarb

Pineapple

Raspberries

Watermelon

Persimmon

Ascerola

Nectarines

85% of Enzymes are destroyed in cooking.

Sources of Vitamin F

Flaxseed Oil*

Evening Primrose Oil*

Borage Oil*

Black Current Oil*

Fish Oil*

Safflower Oil

Olive Oil

Sources of Vitamin K

Alfalfa*

Safflower oil

Green and leafy

vegetables

*indicates sources

available in pill form

necessary to cure

deficiency.

Request for Assistance

Name_____

Diagnosis (if known)_____

I hereby request that recommendations be dowsed for_____

(me/name of relative/friend) from the Universal Force.

_____

(signature)

Mail completed form **along with a self-addressed, stamped envelope to**

Nutrition From the Spirits
P.O. Box 248
Louisville, NE 68037

978-0-595-47711-1

0-595-47711-9